I0130264

IT HURTS

Subhasis Das is an IT professional, a music enthusiast and a fanatic cricket follower. *IT Hurts* is his third novel.

Mahi Singla, a LLB graduate, co-owns a fashion boutique and calls herself a coffeeholic and a SRK devotee.

By the same authors

SUBHASIS DAS

Bowled and the Beautiful: A Cricketer's Love Story
Mom Says No Girlfriend

MAHI SINGLA

12 Hours

I.T. HURTS

SUBHASIS DAS
MAHI SINGLA

RUPA

Published by
Rupa Publications India Pvt. Ltd 2014
7/16, Ansari Road, Daryaganj
New Delhi 110002

Sales Centres:

Allahabad Bengaluru Chennai
Hyderabad Jaipur Kathmandu
Kolkata Mumbai

Copyright © Subhasis Das 2014

This is a work of fiction. Names, characters, places and incidents are either the
product of the author's imagination or are used fictitiously,
and any resemblance to any actual persons, living or dead,
events or locales is entirely coincidental.

All rights reserved.
No part of this publication may be reproduced, transmitted,
or stored in a retrieval system, in any form or by any means,
electronic, mechanical, photocopying, recording or otherwise,
without the prior permission of the publisher.

ISBN: 978-81-291-2481-4

First impression 2014

10 9 8 7 6 5 4 3 2 1

The moral right of the author has been asserted.

Printed at Repro Knowledgecast Limited, Thane

This book is sold subject to the condition that it shall not,
by way of trade or otherwise, be lent, resold, hired out, or otherwise circulated,
without the publisher's prior consent, in any form of binding or cover other
than that in which it is published.

*To all guitarists, artists, actors,
astronauts, cricketers and writers
who ended up being engineers.*

Contents

Beyond the Blues

*H*e stood in front of me, looking like the monster in the nightmares I used to have as a child. He was almost a foot taller than me, bald and black. His arms were the size of my thighs, only well toned. His palms were hard as rock and big enough to grip a football and squash it like a banana. His shiny muscular physique would have put even Hercules to shame. Those big eyes spelt terror and that cruel smile would have been enough to make people piss in their pants. He was designed to kill. He was eyeing me like a hungry lion eyes a baby gazelle. Holy crap! And it wasn't about points, it was a knockout match. Double crap!

I wondered whether he had underestimated his opponent or was just being over confident. On my part, I got myself into the shell position, covering my face with my gloves. He was a true professional; I was sure that he would aim and hit wherever it hurt most. And I would not be able to resist his blows with my clumsy defense. I realized this as soon as he tried to break in with a few quick punches to my head. Attack is the best defense, but under the circumstances, that seemed like a bad idea. He had taken his victory for granted and this actually showed in his approach. He danced all around the ring, waving his hands about and throwing out air kisses. The crowd reacted spontaneously, making him go wild. Of course, I couldn't fight with him as a brawler; one wrong move from me could change his attitude and could prove to be my death knell. It was all about a punch, one perfect hit timed perfectly with all my power. I wanted him to tire of my outside-fighter tactics, and so I kept stalling for time, looking for an opportunity. And when I found one, he was visibly irritated by my quick and sharp counter strike and seemed to be in a hurry to end the game. He had come too close, belting out powerful jabs with both hands, only to give me my chance. I tilted my head back and he missed. His hands weren't guarding his face anymore, and before he had time to think about anything, I shocked him with an upper cut straight on the chin, delivered with all my power, followed by a hard hook to the side of his head with my other hand. The right upper cut followed by a left hook is always a deadly combination, and the devil fell down in the ring, not able to rise after that.

I threw my hands up in the air and jumped, screaming to celebrate my hard-won victory, but the crowd booed me down. Bloody Americans! They just couldn't take defeat. But who cared. I wasn't fighting for them, nor was it something between me and the devil that lay still in front of me. It was a battle between me and my conscience. More appropriately, a release of all the aggravation and fury that had accumulated in my mind. Actually, our greatest battles are the ones we fight with our own minds; for me, this was just one of those, and I had won.

I switched on my cell phone while walking out of the changing room. There was a message from Subho—*We won!* I checked the date, it was 2 April. So finally, we were World Champions after twenty-eight years, and I guessed, I was the last Indian on earth to have found out. I smiled. As I drove off in my Porsche, I tuned in to an Indian radio station to get updates and save myself from public embarrassment. The World Cup meant a lot to Indians. People had come out on the streets with banners and posters of the men in blue, shouting slogans like Jai ho, Chak de. It was a pleasant surprise to see such a celebration for an Indian victory on American soil. It was difficult to believe that I was driving on the streets of New Jersey and not New Delhi. I wondered whether back home in India, we would have been so generous as to allow outsiders to carouse and flaunt their victory.

As expected, my people back in our den were bleeding blue too. The party was at its peak and everyone was invited. The hall was a complete mess, nothing to be found in its usual place. The mattresses from the bedroom were spread out on the floor, pillows were scattered everywhere, and bedcovers had been used to darken the windows. Our stock in the fridge was gone; I could see empty beer bottles rolling, littering the floor. The place smelt of garlic and tomato sauce, clear signs that they had been surviving on Maggi and pizzas for weeks now. They had last slept on 31 March, and yet nothing could deter their spirits today. Subho flipped through the news channels that were repeatedly airing match clippings and celebrations back in India; these were to hog prime time for days to come, to be watched elatedly, again and again by everyone. As everyone gathered at my place did. They were so engrossed that none of them even noticed me coming in. I made my way to my room to take a shower, and half an hour later, when I returned, they were still exactly as I had left them. All eyes firmly glued to the television.

'I promise, I won't even touch the World Cup, but please God, make me Virat Kohli for tonight,' Subho exclaimed, watching the team taking their victory lap.

'I guess Gautam will not like your request, dude!' Ali smirked.

'I heard it!' I cut in, and everyone turned towards me in surprise.

'Hey! You're here,' the blonde shrieked. I didn't really remember her name. They all appeared the same to me. But this one, Subho had told me, had a big crush on me. She worked in our office.

She ran towards me and hugged me tight. 'We won! We won...' she whispered excitedly in my ears.

Why did she care? I wondered whether she knew it was cricket and not football. The expression on my face must have passed on the message to the others because a unanimous hysterical laugh broke out. I pushed her aside, looking at her thin frame, thinking to myself, maybe we Indians had invented the zero, but that doesn't mean we like zero figures.

'What happened to your lips?' she pointed at the cut on my lips.

'Well...I had a romp of a session in bed last night.' That line turned her off and she moved away.

'By the way, he got out cheaply today. You must be happy *na*?'

Ali teased. But one furious glare from me and his small smile, that had been expanding apprehensively, vanished altogether. Ali never dared to take the name, it was always a 'he' when I'm around.

'Hey! To hell with that. The news is that we got the appointment and you people need to leave this week itself.' That was Moody, and she meant me and Subho.

I frowned. 'Why me?'

'Well, we have already had a lot of discussion about that in the past,' she replied.

'But…'

'Listen, Gautam,' Subho intervened. 'The brightest future will always be based on a forgotten past. You can't get on well in life until you let go of past failures and heartaches. And this time, it's just not about you; it's about us.' He patted my back.

I thought about his words for a second; he was right. If not for me, I had to go for their sake, because I owed them. Big time.

'I will go,' I nodded, and Moody smiled. She smiled at just about everything.

∽

I fiddled with my phone, wondering whether I should tell my parents that I was coming to India. Actually, I still didn't want to go; at least not until I completely got over my past. I still didn't know where exactly I was heading; nothing had really helped me. Even after months of isolation, gallons of alcohol, loads of work and some crazy boxing thrown in, I still felt the same way, and I knew my trip to India would only worsen my case. She still ruled my mind, and the harder I tried to forget her, the more my craving for her grew.

Something crossed my mind, and I haplessly searched through my cupboard but just couldn't find what I was looking for. I stopped and closed my eyes, trying to visualize it, and at once, I knew exactly where it was. I opened the drawer and there it was! The little friendship card, lying in the same angle in the same corner where I had dumped it, a year ago. It was the first thing she had given me, after her phone number. I picked up the card—it had two teddy bears dancing on the cover—and I opened it slowly. To the left was the outline of her lips, she had applied lipstick and kissed it at my request. I could still feel her fragrance lingering in the card. On the right it read: *Life is a big party with friends like you around.*

Life wasn't a party anymore; calling it hell would be an understatement. I didn't even remember the last time I had a genuine smile on my face. Fun was an antonym to my personality. People in my office called me 'the dummy'. Life was merely a routine…I hadn't always been this cynical in life. I was once 'Mr Sunshine'. Actually, all I had wanted to do was to run away from her, but in the process, I had lost myself completely. *I hate you for making me love you.*

My phone was playing out the full ringtone for the third time, I realized. Mom was calling. Why the urgency, I wondered. She knew very well that if I wasn't willing to talk, I'd not pick up anyhow. Yes, I could be that rude sometimes. Anyway, I reckoned Subho must have informed her about our arrival.

'Hello!' I accepted the call, and before she could reply, I said, 'Yes, Mom! I'm coming.'

In the Pursuit of Ecstasy

A week later...

I was seated on the stage, yawning for the umpteenth time. We were at a conference arranged by a politician, to felicitate us on our achievements. A considerably huge crowd had turned up. Press, youngsters, kids, a few friends and relatives—all those gathered there made me feel that it was actually something important. Well, you see, back in India, I was quite an item. Since the time we got here, almost every kind of media had featured us. We got numerous calls and emails asking for interviews and shows, but we preferred to be away from the glamour. However, someone had approached through Dad, and I couldn't say no. But then, all this lights, camera and attention! Wasn't all this a bit too much for me, I thought.

Subho, perhaps, was used to it and enjoying it, since he was a published author. He was on the dais, giving a speech that sounded no less than an election campaign speech of some great politician. Not that he had prepared and practiced it last night, but this guy actually knew what to speak, and where. In his own amazing way, he had just announced our arrival in the corporate world—we were there not to stay or grow, we had come to rule. Whoa! He received a grand applause from the audience as he finished and walked back to his seat. But now it was my turn. Shit!

'Hello, everyone!' I greeted them. As the mike squeaked at its loudest, my confidence dropped a few hundred feet. I wondered why this always happened to me. But then, I've always also taken it valiantly. And this day was no different.

'Mr Deshmukh! Tell us how you're actually feeling?'

'Well, call me Gautam! That would be cool. And about your question, I am really feeling rather nervous and scared.'

The audience laughed at my answer.

'I'm serious.'

They stopped laughing.

'You see, I am here to inspire people, maybe act as a role model or something, but trust me, I'm the last person on earth to make a good role model. You know what I actually wanted to be as a kid? You must ask my dad.'

Everyone turned to look at my dad, who wore his hallmark smile, recalling my childhood days.

'I wanted to be Spiderman, but then I thought we don't have those kind of tall buildings down here. Also, I might get tangled in the electric wires.'

There was a strange silence after this.

'I am expecting you to clap.'

And promptly, they all laughed and clapped.

'So Gautam, tell us about your new venture.'

'OK. Now, there's a question I would love to answer. Our new venture is all about 3D tele-presence. In simple language, you could actually beam your friends in 3D while chatting, like in the movies. This technology will let you interact with 3D holograms of your friends in real time. Movies and TV are already moving to 3D, and as 3D and holographic cameras get more sophisticated and miniaturized to fit into cell phones, you will be able to interact with photos, browse the Web and chat with your friends in entirely new ways. The technique uses light beams scattered from objects and reconstructs a picture of that object; the technique is similar to how your eyes visualize your surroundings.' I stopped talking and saw that my speech had left my audience clueless. I realized that the concept of 3D still applied only to Hollywood sci-fi flicks. Looking at the blank faces in front of me, I reckoned I had lost a few of my fans. 'Umm…For people into distance relationships, our venture will definitely bring your loved ones closer, virtually, if not physically. And with your support, we are soon hoping to break into the Forbes list of billionaires.'

There was another round of applause and by now, I was getting a bit embarrassed.

'Sir!' A hand shot up in the audience.

'Gautam!' I insisted.

'Yeah! I'm a computer science student and love studying coding, technology and all that stuff, but then, when I hear about recession, job cuts, long office hours and all, it freaks me out.'

'Well, my dear friend, since you said that you love coding, I want to point out a glitch in what you're saying. IT is not the only victim of recession. Everything around you is affected, even your onion prices. We should soon add recession to the list of natural calamities.'

'I mean, isn't IT unstable?' he argued.

'You're now talking like my Grandma. You see, I really have a tough time when she asks me what my company makes. I will tell you a story. When I went to stay with my Grandma after my final engineering exams, she was thrilled to see me; after all, I was the first person in my family to have earned that degree. I remember she was building a new house. She brought out the architectural plan for the house and asked me to explain it. I told her that I had studied IT and not civil. The next day, I was sitting with her in the kitchen and her mixer-grinder broke down. She asked me to repair it and I told her that I wasn't an electronics guy. In the evening, when we went out and her car stopped in the middle of the road, again she turned to me! This time, I told her that I wasn't a mechanical or automobile engineer. She was truly stunned by this point. She asked me what I had done in college for four years. So I took her to my room and showed her my laptop, but she was like, "This is it?! All this impression we have about IT, and this is it?" I sat with her that day and explained to her what IT actually is.

'In our country, success is measured in terms of money, so I said that the world's richest guy, Bill Gates, is an IT guy. The world's youngest billionaire, Mark Zuckerberg, is also an IT guy. Perhaps, we Indians are not known for our spices or silk anymore, but we're now leaders in IT. Moreover, these days, IT is a part of almost everything that a normal human being does in his life. Virtually every business relies on technology and computer systems. From retail companies to the manufacturing of planes, from pharmaceuticals to mobile recharging. All of them need people to support, manage, assist in creating competitive advantage and protecting their information systems and data. The positions that provide all of those services to businesses comprise the many career choices in IT.

'But if you ask an IT geek who has been passionate about computers right from the days of floppy disks, then my dear friend, for anyone looking for a fun, exciting and growing career option, I would recommend careers in the Information Technology field. I agree that IT hurts for the reasons you gave, but IT rocks too, in its own way.'

The audience responded enthusiastically.

'Thank you very much!' I beamed. It was finally over.

Dad had informed me that one of my school teachers was to attend the function, and that she wanted to meet me afterwards. Although I was tired, I was more than eager to meet Mrs Dasgupta, my English teacher, who I could see was making her way towards me.

'Hello Gautam!' She greeted me with her trademark warm smile. She now looked much older than the teacher I remembered, but her charming personality was the same.

'Hello Ma'am! How are you?'

'I am fine, and I can see that you're doing very well.'

'Thanks Ma'am! I hope the programme was good.'

'Of course! I was surprised at your approach, I admit. You've changed so much. Where has my calm and sincere little Gautam gone?'

'He has grown up and learnt to take life as a man,' I replied.

'Wow! That was smart. We oldies need to accept your style. How do you youngsters say it—*youngistani*? We need to adopt that attitude. Anyway, Gautam, I'm happy for you.'

'Thank you, Ma'am.'

'How is Riya? I heard that she is in the US too.'

'Yeah.' I knew my response was cold. It still hurt after all this time. 'Why didn't she come with you?'

'Well, Ma'am! She is busy with her work, I guess.' I tried to hide my feelings.

'That's really good to hear. So you both stay in the same place?'

'No, I am in New York and she is somewhere in Florida.'

'She was always my favourite, an amazing child. I have something for her. Please give it to her the next time you meet her.' And she opened her handbag and took out a copy of *Heidi*, Riya's favourite story. It was, perhaps, the first novel she had ever read. Back in school, it was to be my library project while hers was *Black Beauty*. But she had completed mine first. And ever since then, she had always loved reading all kinds of books.

I stood there feeling restless, as Ma'am continued talking about Riya. Memories flooded my mind. The gaping hole was still there in my heart. I still cared for her and missed her, but I didn't love her anymore. Now, she just reminded me of someone who had taken her place in my life, the one person who actually brought me back to life after Riya had left me bleeding.

'Sorry Ma'am, I can't take this book. I've not been in touch with Riya for a long time.'

She didn't question me further. Maybe that's what age gives you, a quiet maturity to understand what is not said or maybe the pain in my eyes conveyed itself to her. I left for my car without taking the book.

I was about to reach the main gate when somebody called me. I turned back; a merry little chubby kid was running towards me.

'I liked your speech very much. I have seen you on TV. Truly, when I grow up, I just wanna be like you.'

'Bad idea, dude! Being Gautam is like being single all life. No love, no girlfriend. Only depression. Tell me now, do you want to become like me?'

He shook his head in disappointment. I bent down to match his height and peered into his eyes.

'Take my advice, don't be Gautam. Be Dhruv and rock this world.'

'You know my name?' he looked amazed.

I nodded, 'I saw that on your ID card.'

'You're so cool,' he smiled, and gave me a tight *jaadu ki jhappi*.

∽

We talked, discussed, argued and finally agreed. We signed papers, shook hands and exchanged smiles; the deal was done at last. Our company had pursued this for a long time and it had actually taken the hell out of us over the last few months. We had worked hard during the day and worked harder at nights. No holidays, no weekends. We had made one common time-table which we all followed strictly. However, twenty-four hours of the day seemed too short to implement it, so we compromised on everything—sleep, lunch, dinners, bath, cigarettes, shopping, porn, rest and peace. We went home only to change clothes. Our daily chores were done during breaks from work.

Indian sponsors are a real hard nut to crack. No matter what, wireless technology or the ATM machine concept wasn't respected here and had to be sold to Americans for peanuts. Now, we're making America rich by buying from them what was once made by our own people. But we are eccentric, we are different, we are incredible, we are the Super Six. We ignored that extra money and put in extra effort to make sure that our country was proud of us.

'Don't tell me you don't smoke,' Mr Saxena, one of our sponsors, reacted as I courteously refused cigarettes.

'Why so?' I asked.

'Smoking is so common among you IT geeks,' he said sarcastically.

'Really? Do I look like a geek?' I had barely said anything to attract attention while Mr Saxena was gaping at me skeptically.

'Actually, somebody said I'm very cute and I lose the charm holding that little thing between my fingers!' I smirked. It actually took a few moments for the people around to understand my joke; but what followed was a sea of sophisticated corporate smiles on everyone's faces and relief on Subho's face. My ways always scared him!

But I had just pulled out the wrong card. An endless stream of thoughts swam in my mind after that; I was so restless that I felt as if I were suffocating. Memories of her took over my head and all my senses went blank. I excused myself and hurried to the balcony. I gulped in fresh air by the gallon, leaning heavily against the railings of the forty-storey building, holding on tight. I knew I could not get over it on my own. The pain was growing with every second and I didn't want to screw things up. I took out my little bottle of anti-depressants and swallowed one. I recalled a line I had read somewhere.

That's the thing about pain, it demands to be felt.

'Bro! Take this.' Subho passed me a glass of water. I hadn't noticed but he had been standing behind me all the while.

'I shouldn't have come back to India. It hurts a lot,' I said.

'Dude! It's not about you alone. We all share this dream and you know well enough, that when it comes to talking, you're just the best,' he paused here to check how I was feeling, then went on. 'Be strong, it's been more than a year now. Long time. Face the reality and get over it.'

'I still love her,' I replied.

'Then go and meet her. Our flight is only in the evening,' he said and left.

The tablet had done its bit; the giddiness was gone and I was feeling better. I lifted my head and looked up at the skyline of my city, amchi Mumbai. Not much had changed in a year. A few tall buildings, some extra flyovers, a bit of pseudo greenery, but not quite Shanghai. That was yet a distant dream. Mumbai was still dirty, rowdy and crowded, but even so, it was lively and lovely. Overflowing with energy. It had given me a few incredible memories, it had given me my life. This is where we had met, talked, loved, kissed, fought and then separated forever. A part of me had died after that and I was still searching within, for the old Gauti. Ananya's Gauti. My vision seemed clouded over by now with tears filling up my eyes, I quickly wiped them with the back of my palm and tried a half smile. This was all I had been doing over the last entire year.

∽

I wondered whether he had actually brought me there on purpose. Twice, I asked him about it, but Subho just said that he had wanted to drive through the scenic Worli sea link, and he seemed very amazed as he dodged cars speeding at 100 miles per hour on that super bridge. He had an American driving license and I wanted to tell him that driving in India was totally different, but I liked this carefree side I was seeing in him. He drove us to Bandra Fort.

It's true that when you're single, you see happy couples and when you're a couple, you see happy singles. However, I had my own memories of this place to cherish; I came here once with Ananya. Actually, there are certain moments from my life that I'd like to put on continuous replay. But I guess what makes them so beautiful and so memorable is knowing that I can never have them back again. I felt the old familiar urge rising in me. I desperately needed to see her, to kiss her and hug her, or to simply hear her voice. I couldn't resist the feeling any more; I took out my phone and dialled 09329136996. I had deleted her number from my phone a long time ago but I couldn't remove it from my heart even after a whole year had passed. I guess I would never be able to.

CDMA numbers always took time to connect, and with each beep, my heart was pounding hard. I wondered whether she still used the same number. It did get connected, but as always, it was busy. I stayed on line wondering what I would say to her after all this time. Would she even talk to me? Maybe she would shout at me again. After a while, I disconnected and put the phone back into my pocket.

We left soon after; we had a flight to catch. On the way back, I checked my phone. It had a message—*Whoz dis? Please call.* I ignored the message, perhaps because Subho was right next to me or perhaps that same old male ego came in the way. And then she called me, but again I ignored her. Once, twice, thrice. Finally, she stopped calling. Once we reached the airport, I hurried to the washroom and checked my phone but it was blank. Suddenly I wanted to talk but was in two minds now; all those questions came back. I knew for a fact that she too didn't care.

We found out that our flight was delayed by some three hours due to bad weather. Was it just a coincidence or was it some kind of signal? I didn't know. Something was to happen, whether good or bad. I remained silent for the longest time and my behaviour was enough for Subho to pick up a vibe. So, to avoid facing him, I debated whether I should check my mails. I opened Facebook instead.

I had blocked her from my list but knew that she would never do the same. Maybe she still didn't know how to do it. Facebook was like rocket science to her. She was quite dumb in such matters. Whether I saw her or not, I knew she would be the same lovable, cute and stupid Ananya, with no chance of improvement, but still the sweetest part of my heart. I was confident about her because nothing much seemed to have changed in her profile, not even the display picture. And more importantly, she was still 'Single'. Or at least, her Facebook profile said so.

Unwillingly, I sent her a friend request. I wanted to see more of her, her friends, her profile and her wall. I wanted to know everything about her. But then, she hardly ever logged in. And moreover, I didn't want to take this pain back with me to America; this was a closed chapter. I went back to cancel the request but somebody's hand on my shoulder stopped me. I turned around, it was Subho.

'So you'll not change!'

'It's nothing. I was just checking,' I defended myself.

'Checking what? Dude! As if I don't know, you called her too.'

'I'm sorry.'

'There is no need for this. Gautam, I don't want to see you like this. If you want, you can call her, but change this bloody expression on your face.'

'I thought you would be angry.'

'I give a damn! I just want you to be happy, with or without her. It's your life, your call. I never had a problem with her. You broke up with her. It was your decision. Staying away from your country, your home, your family and your friends won't help. You've not changed even a bit in this entire period, she still means everything to you. You can't run away from reality like that. You still love her,' he yelled at me and I looked down at my feet sheepishly.

'We've got a lot of time, you can go and meet her,' he added after a long silence.

'No. I just want to hear her voice once,' I said.

'Your wish.' He shrugged his shoulders.

I dialled her number. It rang for a while; she always took a hell of a lot of time to pick up. With every passing ring, my confidence wore thin, and when she finally said a hello, I went weak in my knees. She began shouting after a point and the only thing I could do was to take a deep breath. She was still the same—my daunting and demanding Ananya, whom I used to talk to ten times a day and talk rubbish, but today, I just couldn't utter a word. I disconnected the call.

'Hello!' she shouted, when I called her again after some time, but again, I found no words to say.

'Gauti, is that you?' she caught me.

'Yes…it's me…Ananya!' I was actually shocked.

'Gauti, will you talk to me properly? What's wrong with you?' she demanded.

What's wrong with me? I was never expecting such a reaction. Say *missed you, waiting for you, love you* or the opposite of all those things like *go to hell, hate you* or simply *fuck off*. I mean, I had called her after over a year and she was so casual about it! Hadn't my absence bothered her at all? But then she had recognized me without a word. 'How do you know it's me?' I asked. I knew that she still cared for me, she always did.

'Baby, it's only you who used to give blank calls even earlier,' she said. *Baby!* I liked that. I knew she was smiling now.

'Sorry, Ananya!'

'Shut up now! Tell me how are you? And where the hell are you? It's been a long time since we talked.'

'More than a year.' I paused and blurted out, 'I missed you a lot.'

'I missed you too,' her voice became heavy.

'I am in India for some work. My flight back got delayed for a few hours, so I thought of calling you.'

'So…' She tried to get the better of me but by no means was I going to let her win.

'Nothing. Bye.'

'Gauti, wait. I want to meet you.'

Zero Percentile

Three years ago...

I didn't want to go back to Pune, I wanted to join the company that same week, but the HR guys had not yet called me for the medical test. I had been trying her number since morning, but it went unanswered. It was already 10.30 a.m. and she was still not at her desk, how disgusting was that! However, I continued calling, and after what seemed like ages, she picked up.

'Hello!'

'Hi, Madam! This is Gautam Deshmukh.'

'Who?'

'Madam, the new joinee.'

'OK! Let me check on my system,' she interrupted. I waited for her to get back. 'Yeah! Tell me, Gautam.'

'Madam, actually I called you to find out about the medical test.'

'I told you, I will mail you the details. Have some patience,' and she cut the call.

Now, I had just one alternative, to lie to Mom that I had joined, but I didn't like the thought of it. I always get caught out, I'm a bad liar. But then, no way was I going to go back home. I had left behind a lot of things and I didn't have the courage to face them anymore. I wanted some solitude, some peace. *Maybe I should switch off my phone till I get the joining date.* Bad idea! My parents showing up here, that was the last thing I wanted.

*Got my eyes on you, won't you bring that back to me...*My phone sang aloud. A call from HR

'Hi! This is Bhakti. May I know who's this?'

'Madam, it's me, Gautam.'

'Who Gautam?'

'Madam, Gautam Deshmukh. We just talked a few minutes ago.'

'Really?'

'Yes. Well, I am the new joinee.'

'OK! Let me check on my system.' Seriouly. HR people *are* that dumb. They don't have their brains in place, their brains are in their systems.

'Oh! I got you. Dude, you called me twelve times.'

'Thirteen. You picked up at my thirteenth attempt.'

'Why, man? What's the matter?'

'I need this job desperately.'

'You already got it, right?'

'No. I mean, I want to join at the earliest. Please, on this Monday itself.'

'Well, I'm sorry. I've talked to the people at the medical center, they are fully booked. No more appointments for the week.'

'Do you have their number?' I asked with intensity in my voice. This little question actually was to change my life forever. I sometimes wish I hadn't gone that mad that day. I should have lied to my Mom, gone back home for a week, or simply called them here. But then, my destiny had already been written, you see.

'Why?'

'I'll request them myself.'

'Boy! You're driving me crazy,' she yelled at me.

'Please,' I begged, and the magical word worked again.

'OK!' she agreed. 'Let me check on my system.'

❦

I got an appointment finally, after Bhakti had pestered them a lot on my behalf. However, I learned the reason she had been insisting on another day, only as I entered the medical centre. It was an All Ladies day. Any other day, I would have felt really lucky but that day, I was rather embarrassed to be there, so I took a seat at the far back, and wished for it to get over quickly.

And then, I saw her.

It can't be true! Riya is gone, USA, better life, more fun, and no loser boyfriend (read me), I thought. But then the same beautiful face, arched brows, almond eyes and that sparkling smile that created those deep dimples. *She came back? For me? She loves me; which meant she lied to me the other day. She was just testing me. It was a prank, or better still, just a nightmare.* All these unreal possibilities were popping up in my mind endlessly. Thoughts clogged my mind like programme codes, and I could feel myself going mad, gaping at her movements throughout. Finally, it hit me. She wasn't Riya for sure. Riya never wore green; she hated this colour, madly. Who was she then? Her name was Ananya Singh, I checked in her form as she passed me a pen. Her clone or her lost twin sister. I didn't yet know but I wanted to find out.

Her number was called out, she rose and went in. I followed her.

'Excuse me! Where are you going?' the receptionist inquired.

'Well...' I gave her a sheepish look and mumbled, 'Toilet...I want to go to the toilet.' I had just made it worse. All the ladies sitting there smirked at me, highly amused.

'Washroom actually,' I tried to correct my English.

'Then take this jar with you and fill it,' she snapped at me while the rest of them giggled. Embarrassment at its best! I had nothing left to say, and no choice. I picked up the jar and rushed to the men's room. I didn't know where she had disappeared, and now, I didn't care either.

To be frank, I was anxious to see the colour of my urine sample. A blood test was to follow. I was worried because some time ago, my life had been a complete mess. I had gone through a phase when I was down all the time, lost to reality. I couldn't get through a single day without parties and night outs. I drank too much, smoked all the time, and also did drugs. I prayed none of that would come out in the medical report. I really needed this job, it was my only chance to get over my horrific past. I wanted to build a new present, leave behind all those dark memories.

'Relax! It's just a little needle,' the nurse bawled at me, seeing my expression. I turned away. My mystery girl was standing just behind me, blushing. Maybe because of me! Or so I thought to myself. That smile, or to be precise, those dimples made me think again. She was driving me crazy. I made up my mind to talk to her later.

I soon got my chance. The nurse went out with our blood samples, leaving us both alone in that small room. What an opportunity! But then, I was such a dork and so shy, I never knew how to take chances, and from what I had seen, normally, girls didn't take initiatives. So we just remained silent. It was an awkward situation; we looked around all over the room full of medicines, needles, jars and all kinds of stuff fit to make anyone sick, and when our eyes met, we exchanged blank looks and *not-again* smiles. It continued that way for some time. I didn't know a thing about her, yet I was desperate to talk to her. But I only managed some strange expressions while she completely ignored me, took her phone out and started messaging her friends. Later, I would find out that this was her habit, she always did it to distract her mind. Every day, morning to evening! When she was alone or bored. And they all replied to her messages and made her smile. That was her way to make her presence felt in their life, until they got used to her and couldn't live without her. She was that cruel, I was to find out. So anyway, sitting there in that room alone with her, I was pissed off and I gave up trying to begin a conversation. I had my own toys to play with. I pulled out my iPad, the latest model.

'Excuse me!' she cried. If not me, my gadgets did get noticed.

'Yes,' I grunted, still looking at the screen. NFS rocks!

'Please listen to music on your earphones,' she requested in a stern voice. She didn't like being ignored, I thought to myself.

'Well!' I paused my game. 'It's not music; I'm playing a game, NFS. You see, it's a motion sensor.'

Yes, I can be irritatingly over-informative sometimes. After all, I'm an engineer.

'So?' she said, in a way that sounded like *fuck off.* That was really rude.

If someone gives you shit, give back two buckets of shit. That's what I believe strongly, and follow even more strongly. But that day was different; I put my iPad back in my bag and stayed silent. After all, she was a girl and moreover, the craving was mine. I wanted to be nice to her. I still wanted to talk to her somehow. But what followed was more of the same awkward silence between us. She was done with her SMSs and her cell phone didn't offer too many other options.

'Can you pass the pen?' Her tone wasn't polite. I still gave her the pen, beaming.

No response.

She took the pen, pulled out a paper and tried to sketch. The most common one everybody does, a face of a girl—squint eyes, crooked nose, big lips, hair all over. She was quite bad at it, and she knew it very well too, yet she was expecting some compliment. I guessed that from the way she looked at me out of the corner of her eyes. I chose to ignore her. I didn't want to disappoint her with my bluntness.

Some more silence. 'Hello!' she said finally, as our eyes met again. The ignoring technique always worked on girls.

'Hi!' I smiled.

'I'm Ananya. Ananya Singh.'

'I'm Gautam Deshmukh.'

'Nice to meet you.'

'Same here. Do you know Riya?' I didn't want to miss out on this chance to find out.

'What? Who Riya? No!' she was confused.

'Are you from Pune?' I continued, somewhat confident about the possibilities.

'No. I'm from Panvel,' she seemed appalled now.

'Which department?' I went on.

She gave me a stern glare, I hung my head.

'Accounts,' she replied. 'You?'

'QC. Quality Control.'

'You're an engineer right? And also a fresher I guess,' she interrupted.

'Yes but how do you know?'

'It shows,' she said. Was that a compliment or a taunt?

'You are also an engineer?'

'Na. M.Com. Four years experience,' she answered boldly. So 'fresher' wasn't a taunt or a compliment, it was an insult.

'Hey! I'm not a fresher really. I handled my Dad's business for two years. You know Deshmukh Finance?' I did have something to flaunt.

She narrowed her eyes, made a face like an angry child. I made up my mind not to bother her the rest of the time we needed to spend there.

'Ananya, you may leave. We will let you know the results,' the nurse informed her.

She picked up her stuff and got up. I didn't dare to even look at her.

'So see you then. Bye,' she said. This time she sounded a bit gentle.

'Ya, bye,' I beamed. She walked slowly, lazily. The sketch was still held in her hand. I knew she was still expecting a compliment.

'By the way, nice sketch,' I said out loud when she had reached the door.

She turned to look at me with childlike glee, and that smile bowled me over.

∽

Four days since I had joined, and I was already bored. More so because I had nothing to do. I was done with the initial formalities, bank accounts, documentation and all kind of inductions. My training was to start once other newcomers joined, which was still two weeks away. My new machine had not yet been delivered and I was given a seat next to my reporting manager, Mr Muthu Kumar, or rather Mr *Panauti*. He wasn't really a bore; he was a boar, a wild one.

Though my company had one of the coolest campuses, I hardly knew anyone one to hang out with. I had already spent a few days in the office but hadn't made any friends yet. Perhaps, I didn't want to. But there was this one person I still wanted to meet—Ananya Singh. I hadn't forgotten her. Actually, from my very first day, I was on a hunt for her but she was nowhere to be seen. I had searched everywhere—inductions, food courts, hangouts, parking, bus stop, station, and even the corporate telebook, but all in vain. Lastly, I decided to go to the medical centre and get her contact details, but knew I wouldn't be able to give them a proper reason, and even if I did, what would I say to her about how I got her number. And more importantly, why I called her.

I gave up.

∽

Unlike most other days, I wasn't actually strolling around. I was very tired of doing nothing in the office and wanted to go home, straight to bed. But I missed my regular train by a second because I was too lazy to walk faster. So I waited, eagerly scanning the railway schedule on my phone screen to check the timing of the next available train. There were fifteen minutes to go. I sat down on a bench and leaned back to rest my head. I had almost dozed off, when somebody poked me in the arm.

'I guess she is calling you,' he said.

I looked up to see a girl waving at me. I couldn't see her clearly though, I was still somewhat dazed. She stood on the other side; I walked to the edge of the platform. *Ananya? Was I dreaming?!* I couldn't believe it! I looked around; it was just me and that fat ass who had woken me up. It was me, she was calling out to!

'Hi!' I screamed and waved back with a big smile, of course.

'Hello!' she couldn't match my voice, not because she was a girl, but because I was the one more excited.

'I can't hear you,' I shouted even louder, enough to turn a few heads. Embarrassment! Girls can't take it.

'Wait,' she gestured and in another second, she disappeared in the crowd.

'Gautam, you're such a loser,' I said to myself.

I went back to my comfortable position on the bench and resumed dozing but again, somebody poked me. I wondered why people couldn't mind their own business. I ignored whoever it was jabbing my arm. This time, the person shook my shoulders and I almost slipped from the seat. I regained my balance and turned to glare violently.

Ananya. Standing right in front of me. What was happening?

'Hey!' I grunted.

'Boy, you're so rude,' she said.

'Am I?'

'A lady is standing in front of you and you're relaxing on the bench, pathetic!' I was to learn that she used this word 'pathetic' in almost every line she spoke. *Now that's really pathetic.*

'Oh sorry!' I stood up straight.

'That's OK! I was just kidding.'

'By the way, you almost disappeared after that day.'

'Well, I should say the same for you.'

'Yeah!' She smiled.

'You were there, right?' I pointed to the other side of the platform. 'I came down the subway for you,' she said. *Wow! She came all the way here for me.*

'Actually, you were shouting like hell and people were staring at us. That was really pathetic. So, I thought that it was better to come over here,' she added.

'You stay in Panvel, right?'

'You still remember?' she was amazed.

'Ya. I mean you told me that just some six days ago.'

'Are you *kinda* hitting on me?' she asked outright.

Was I expected to confess? I gave her a blank look.

'I'm just kidding, boy!'

'Hmmm,' I beamed, but that was a close call.

'OK,' she paused, 'where do you stay?'

'Nerul.'

'Wow! Same train and I guess it's time now. I should go ahead near the ladies coach. Give me your number.'

'What?!' That was really spontaneous.

'Your number. Your mobile number,' she clarified. Did I say earlier that girls don't take the initiative? Well, I can be wrong sometimes. Very rare though.

'Actually, I don't remember my number, so you better give me yours and I will give you a missed call.'

I was not playing smart; I honestly didn't recall my own number as I had switched to a new number in Mumbai and had hardly used my phone yet. I wanted to remain somewhat isolated.

She didn't think twice either to give her number, probably because of the approaching train. I dialled her number while she rushed towards her compartment. But hang on! Please check the number you've dialled, said my phone. I checked and counted the numbers. Nine digits. I had missed one. I looked down the platform, the train was already visible near the crossing, but I didn't want to miss her this time. Who knew when we would meet again? I raced in her direction, making my way through the crowd which had gathered to board the train. I didn't know how many people I tumbled into nor did I care for the abuses they yelled at my speeding back. I just ran like a madman. I didn't want to lose her. I was fucking alone in this city.

Once I reached her compartment, I found her standing a little away from the door. She was talking on her phone but I did not have the time or patience to wait for her call to end. She was a bit astonished to see me there and instantly cut the call. Some *Sach* was on the other side of the call, I had heard that much.

'What?' she reacted. Sach called her again, she rejected the call.

'Well, you gave me a wrong number,' I said sheepishly.

'Really?' she said, cutting Sach's third attempt.

I showed her the number.

'Well, add another 9 before the last 6.'

'OK.'

'Ya, now run. The train has arrived,' she said and moved away, melting into the crowd.

I too hurried toward the gents coach and blindly lunged into the sea of humanity, and the rest was taken care of by the generous Mumbaikars. So I was in, thanks to them, without any effort from my side, though I won't say I was positioned very comfortably. But at least I had enough space around me to take my phone out of my pocket. I called her right away, which I knew was quite desperate, but luckily her number was busy. Sach was finally successful, I guessed.

∽

After Riya, the word *life* had become alien to me. Once back from office, I literally had nothing to do. A full time maid took care of all the household chores, so I just wandered around at work till I felt sleepy enough to return to my place. Before I came to Mumbai, I thought of finding myself some roommates. I had heard stories of engineer roommates—two rooms, one bed, five guys, five hundred beer bottles, a million cigarette butts, Maggi for dinner, dirty bed sheets, Pink Floyd all the time—it all sounded cool but then I was yet to find someone like that. Instead, back in office, people seemed rather creepy, I was just another source of competition, and when they talked, they only talked about ratings and package. Talking to them individually, you would know that everyone hated each other, especially if you were a Team Lead. Corporate life is really a bitch!

Anyway, back to my story. I was bored of the malls, I'd never been a shopaholic. I came to check out girls, but then weekdays are not-so-lucky days. I walked to the theatre and there wasn't anything exciting showing, yet I bought a ticket for the movie *Luck*. Of course just to see Shruti Hasan in a bikini, I mean what else did it have to offer. However, here's some advice—if you've broken up recently, then avoid such dud movies; they are the best hangout spot for couples searching for some cozy privacy. Rather than the movie itself, it was such couples seated all over the theatre that pissed me off, and what was really funny was the fact that I kept looking at the right bottom corner of the big screen as if to check the time. I was already settling into the world of corporate etiquette.

Finally, I received a call from Kantabai (my maid) that she was done for the day and was leaving the keys with the security guard. I felt sleepy and left the theatre. I picked up a few things which Kantabai had asked me to buy from Big Bazar and was heading for the parking lot, when I noticed her in the escalator. I wasn't sure it was Ananya, I guessed I was just thinking about her too much, but when I checked closely, it really was her. And she was not alone, there was a guy with her, which gave me a strange pain in the chest as if someone had just stabbed me. Suddenly I just wanted to reach home as soon as possible. But as our escalators crossed, she did notice me and was about to wave at me, but I turned away and rushed to the parking area. I should have known it. She was anyway too pretty to be single. *That guy had to be Sach.*

Back home, I lay on my bed crying. I missed Riya. I always did, because I still loved her. The Ananya episode only added to the pain and made me wonder whether Riya was seeing someone else too. I remained that way all night, alone and crying quietly in the dark. I didn't even remove my shoes, let alone change my clothes. It seemed like everything around me had come to a standstill. I was in a very low mood. No cigarettes, no alcohol, I didn't have the energy to move even once from the bed, and yet, the next morning, I felt some kind of hangover. My head was pounding badly, maybe because I was hungry. The stale food of the previous night was hard to swallow; Kantabai was now habituated to seeing all her efforts gone into the dustbin. I checked my phone. Numerous calls from Mom and Dad, a few messages from friends, and one from Ananya too. I ignored all of them.

I didn't skip office and instead got there well in time, yawning before my PC. What else could I do? Forget about Facebook, Rediffmail was also blocked at work, and nobody knew me yet to mail me on my company ID. My proximity to Muthukumar prevented me from trying my hand at Pinball or Solitaire, and no way was I going to go through the training notes. I wished I hadn't come, not just to office but to Mumbai itself. I understood how hard it was for my parents to let me go, as I saw another call from Dad flashing on my phone. I didn't pick up.

I sent him a message.

I m F9. Slept early yest. Nw in office. Dont call.

I got a message back, not from Dad but from Ananya.

Wassup buddy. I m bored. Wat abt u? Pls reply.

I called her.

'Hey!'

'Hi.' She did sound bored.

'What's up?'

'Nothing re! What about you?'

'No work yet.'

'OK then can we meet? Let's say for a coffee in food court.'

'When?'

'Now.'

'OK. Let me see. I'll call you in five minutes,' I hung up.

Not that I particularly wanted to go out with her, it was more like I was dying to get out of my seat, it didn't matter with whom. And it wasn't that tough to convince Muthukumar. *Meeting HR* is the best excuse for such occasions, and anyway, I hardly existed for anybody there in my office.

She was already waiting for me at the food court. She waved her hand as she saw me coming. I gave a small smile. I wondered what had actually made me so disappointed earlier. I hardly knew her to be jealous or upset about the fact that she had a boyfriend. Was it the enigma of her being Riya that was still bothering me? I knew she wasn't. I hadn't exactly observed it earlier, but she looked a few pounds heavier than Riya. Nor had I noticed before those acne scars on her face; pimples had never dared to touch Riya. And those eyes confirmed it, hers were dark brown; Riya's had a tinge of blue in them, I had actually spent a major part of my life looking into them.

'I guess I saw you yesterday at Nerul Station,' she initiated the conversation, as we sat down with our coffees opposite each other at a table. I had gone all dumb after our initial *hellos*.

'Ya, I saw you too. With him,' I added. For a second, she glared at me and then was back to sipping her coffee.

'Who was he?' I asked. She ignored my question completely. 'Your boyfriend?' I asked again.

'Why should I tell you?' she snapped.

'His name is Sachin, right?'

'What?' She almost spat out a mouthful of coffee in her surprise. No. 'Shocked' is the word. 'How do you know all this?'

'What?' I donned a slick smile but it didn't impress her.

'Just tell me how?' she banged her mug on the table in rage.

'OK, OK.' I narrated everything in terror then, how I had connected the dots.

It was hard to judge from her expression whether she was impressed or angry. She was thinking deeply about something for sure. Maybe about Sachin but I dared not ask her that. I continued playing with my spoon while she finished her coffee.

'Why don't you drink your coffee?' she ordered.

'I don't like coffee.'

'Then why did you take it?'

'For you,' I said, and she returned a stern gaze. I thought if I continued like that, she would slap me for sure. *No more words, pay the bill and run away,* I made a mental note.

'Let me tell you something,' her tone wasn't pleasing, 'if a girl meets a guy that doesn't mean that he is her boyfriend.'

Her blunt words were like a tonic to me. I decided to be careful the next time I interacted with girls.

'By the way, the guy you saw there was Nitin and not Sachin. He is just an old friend and not my boyfriend, OK?'

'Hmm,' I grunted, still not looking at her.

'C'mon it's OK now. I don't like sad faces, cheer up, kid!'

'Stop calling me kid just because I'm a fresher. You see, I'm twenty-four already.'

'Really?' she raised her eyebrow, 'it's still quite young for me. I'm twenty-eight.'

The Delayed Monsoon

Three months later...

'Hello!' Ananya had called me.

'Hey! I was just about to call you,' I said.

'Really? Gauti, you're so bad. You never call me.'

'Do I need to?' Actually, I hardly ever called her when in office, because as I said, I never needed to. I mean, she called me when her system failed, when she walked over to the printer or pantry, when she was in the train, when her boss scolded her, when she felt sleepy, when she wanted to go home, or when she simply wanted to talk to me. And that totalled up to some ten to twelve calls a day, but still our voices carried the same excitement as if we were talking after years.

'Very funny! Actually, I called to inform you that I'm going out with my group. So, don't wait for me today.'

'Well, I'm going out with friends too.'

'Gauti, that's pathetic,' she bawled at me. 'You're not going to do that.' It hardly took any time to spur her into full fury mode. Her temper was always there, sitting on her little nose, ready to burst.

'What? I too have got friends and it's Diwali night, can't I go out? Why do you always feel I'll be after you,' I tried to act cool.

'It's better if you're not,' she snapped at me.

'Anu, you always shout at me. Even today. It's Diwali, damn!' It hurt so much each time she talked like that, but I never told her.

'Happy Diwali, dear. Have fun,' she said. She never apologized.

'Same to you.'

'That's better,' she giggled. 'So, how was your day?'

'It was cool, had lots of fun but missed you.'

'Really? But you seemed so happy with your Mudrika. She was looking pretty today.'

'C'mon, stop it! You know I don't like her that way but she is a great friend.'

'Hmmm,' she sighed. The corporate employee mobile plan had given us such liberty to talk rubbish all day, without paying a penny.

'You were better; you look so beautiful in a sari.'

'Really? How much?'

'What?'

'Tell me how beautiful?' she demanded.

'Well, if I have it my way, I would change the dictionary definition of the word "beautiful" to your name!'

'Wow! That's a great compliment. Thanks,' she blushed. Well, thanks to Facebook, I had scored. That line was Subho's Facebook status.

'You too look good in your traditional outfit.' Her compliments were always flat. She never praised anyone spontaneously to their face.

'By the way, where are you people going?' I asked her casually.

'Gauti!' She screamed, 'You're just too much.'

'Sorry but I'm just worried a bit.'

'I can take care of myself, OK?'

'I know but Gajendra, I don't trust him a bit.'

'Don't think too much. I'll be fine.'

'OK. But don't take any drink from him. Don't get too late and call me as soon as you reach home.'

'Gauti! That's enough, you're irritating me now. Bye,' she hung up. I was still not finished but knew there was no use calling back, she wouldn't listen. Perhaps, she wouldn't even pick up my call in the first place. I didn't want to spoil my mood either, after all it was Diwali night.

∽

It took a lot of effort on my part to convince my friends to go to Thane and not Vashi. Though she didn't tell me, I knew for sure that they would go to the nearby Brass Monkey in Palm Beach Galleria, Vashi. So, by no means I wanted us to cross paths with Ananya's group. But then, Thane was too far for my group, and more importantly, they knew well enough why I was arguing in favour of Thane. They didn't like her. They hated her. They kept telling me that she was a bitch and was just playing around with me.

It was some Night Rider in Thane west, one of those places which were recently upgraded to a pub, after dance bars had been banned in the state. It still wore the signs of its past—a small bar, banal furniture, bad lights and item numbers for music. But at least there were a few girls around, grooving away, which ultimately saved me. Anyway, it was the first time for Subho and Pritam, so they didn't mind anything, but Ali did. 'Damn! Is this what you call a pub?' Ali sounded dismayed, 'the music is so cheap. Look at the crowd, man!' He pointed out a few guys on the dance floor making rowdy moves, as if dancing in Ganpati visarjan. Bloody BPO crowd!

We moved towards the so-called lounge, cut off from the rest of the area by curtains. Well, in its glory days, it did give a feel of heaven. With my group, it was always me who scanned the menu card. I ordered two quarters of RC and chicken. Ali touched nothing. How could someone go to a pub and not drink even water, how strange!

It wasn't as if they were drinking for the first time but Subho and Pritam seemed excited, probably because the place was a pub now and the drinks were neat. And as I filled up their glasses with small pegs, the excitement soon became apprehension, and after downing the drink, they just sat there, aghast.

'It's so hard!' Subho hardly cried for anything.

'What do you expect from a neat drink. It's not orange juice.'

'Whatever!' Subho was still appalled. He ordered a 7up to mix with his drink while Pritam drank a Breezer for the rest of the night. Ali just lazily walked around the place and stood at the bar. 'I guess they don't serve men,' Subho laughed seeing Ali chatting so casually with the bartender. We ignored the comment, pissed off with Ali's homosexual jokes.

'Gautam! There is something you would want to see,' Ali came running.

'No dude! I don't want to see anything with you,' I snapped. Ali's instincts always scared me.

'C'mon dude!' he pulled me from my seat. 'Look there! She is your chick, right?' he pointed at the far corner. It was Ananya with her group. Gajendra too! I hated him. He sucks.

You see when you love someone and you don't know the reason, that's true love. Same way as when you hate someone and you don't know the reason, it's true hatred. Pure. Unadulterated. Hatred. And that's what I felt for him, though Ananya had tried to reason with me many times. I guess it was his bloody awful attire that put him down in my view initially, and eventually, he had crept to the top of my hit list. His teeth had a tinge of black, addicted as he was to tobacco, and lastly, his squint eyes completed the package, giving him a horrible appearance. I wonder if he would really ever need to do anything to his face or body during Halloween, he looked scary all the time!

They were all partying away and their table had everything that would worry me. I did want to intervene but then why should I care, I thought. Her friends, her call, her life. Anyway, she always gave a damn about my words. I ignored her and went back to my table.

'What did you see?' Subho asked. I didn't reply.

'Actually,' Ali chimed in but one furious glare from me and he shut his mouth.

'Ananya.' Subho got it. I nodded and finished my glass in a single gulp.

'She is here,' Ali said.

'Please, I don't want to talk about it. Let's just enjoy the night,' I intervened.

'That's better,' Subho said. 'Cheers!' We toasted our drinks in mid-air but things soon got cold. The gala atmosphere had soured. I had spoiled everyone's mood. A strange silence sank in after that. We quietly went on with our drinks. No fun. No excitement.

Ali left us; he had found his new muse in the bartender. And with Subho and Pritam together, God help you. We hardly exchanged any words, and even if we did, we talked either about past grades or future career aspirations. I would be the last person on earth to give a thought to such topics, I hardly cared. I was in Mumbai just to move on from my past. But the others refused to think beyond their everyday cold war. Their gyan-giving conversations were always meant to end on the big question as to who was the best amongst them. I chose not to get in the way and upset anyone on such a festive occasion. Instead, I stole a glance at the other corner, to where Ananya was sitting.

She had not noticed me yet; besides, she was in her own league. Her table was still bothering me; actually there wasn't a single thing there that could give me relief. No juice or ice-cream, and those soft drinks were there only to dilute alcohol, I was sure. Those crazy moves, funny gestures, silly comments followed by loud laughs—it was all making me feel insane, and if that wasn't enough, they all moved to the dance floor.

It wasn't as if I was jealous of how close she was to her friends, but it hurt me because she never danced with me. I wondered whether this was the same Ananya I had known these past few months, who had been fasting on Mondays for her to-be-husband since the age of ten, and had never ever heard a *Guns and Roses* track. My *desi girl* was just going gaga over a cheesy item number and her whacky moves would have just given *Piggy Chops* a run for her money. What really inspired that devil-may-care attitude in her that night—the occasion, the place, the song or the drink? I grabbed a glass from the waiter who had served them and took a sip.

Antiquity Blue with Spirit. I knew them all, I once drank like pig.

And that pushed the limit for me. I shoved Subho's hand as he tried to stop me and headed straight to the dance floor in full rage. She didn't see me I suppose, but her friends did see me coming and stood between her and me. And like my friends, her friends too didn't like me. They hated me even more and called me a dog, but for different reasons.

'Just stay away. It's between me and Ananya,' I warned them. Subho and Pritam had come to my side by then. No doubt, Pritam was ready to flex his biceps.

'What's the matter?' Ananya pushed her friends. 'Gautam, what are you doing here?' The music had stopped and we stood in the middle of the dance floor, face to face, as the people all around us gaped at us for some entertainment.

'What? What's wrong?' Ananya shouted.

I didn't reply but pulled the glass from her hand, from which she had been drinking all the while.

'It's nothing, it's just a soft drink,' she said.

'Really?'

No way was I going to buy her story; I drank up the rest of it in one go.

Sprite. Only Sprite. Nothing else.

She was furious and stood staring at me.

'What's all this? I don't understand what you're up to?' she yelled, as I looked down at the floor, now embarrassed.

'I'm sorry,' I mumbled. 'I didn't mean to.'

'Whatever!' She paused to have a look around. The damage was already done, so now it actually didn't matter anymore and she continued, 'You're just getting on my nerves. I told you not to follow me.'

'I wasn't following you, OK.' I knew it was my fault but I couldn't bear to see her friends smirking at me.

The male ego. Period.

'I just care for you too much. But you will never understand that.'

'Just go to hell,' she turned away; she almost had tears in her eyes. But the whole situation had hurt me too. I stormed out of the pub. To hell with her and her friends!

It was raining outside. Till today, I wonder sometimes, what was special about that year that the monsoon never seemed to stop. The sky was pouring daggers and the wind tore away at almost everything in its way. It would have been mere stupidity if I had dared to fight back nature's fury with my little umbrella in search of the railway station. Moreover, I didn't even know where it was anymore. I waited under a shop roof for my friends to join me, but when they didn't come along for a while, it did worry me. This was the first time I was in Thane, I didn't know anything about the place. I called Subho, his number was not reachable, nor were Pritam's and Ali's, maybe the thunder shower effect. I thought about going back but the Ananya episode was hurting me. I decided to wait for them outside.

As I kept peering down the lane, hoping for someone to come along, I saw a shadow nearing me. The heavy showers had diminished visibility, yet I knew the person approaching was not the one I was expecting. It was Ananya walking towards me casually, unaffected by the pouring rain. She never carried an umbrella or a raincoat. She loved getting drenched in the rain. Unlike other days, when I never let her carry on with her romance with the rain, I stayed back in the shade that day, just watching her come my way. Her fair and beautiful face still carried some of her fury from the pub; the little smile which had always given me a reason to stay happy was missing. Something bad was to follow, I reckoned. A tight slap perhaps.

'Hi!' she said as she came and stood beside me. I wasn't looking at her.

'Hello!' I greeted coldly.

'Waiting for someone?'

'Hmm,' I sighed. So far, things seemed normal. 'For my friends.'

'They seem to have ditched you,' she smiled mischievously. I glared at her. *Calculus problems are easier to understand than you,* I thought.

'Yeah, looks like that,' I smiled back.

'Any idea how we can return home now?' she said. *WE. She wanted to come with me.*

'You know, I'm the new guy in town.'

'Three months!' she wiggled her fingers, 'You're such a nerd. Well, I know the way to the station, come,' she pulled me by my hand and led me down the street. The rain had weakened now to a mere drizzle.

'Anyway, I'm sorry about tonight,' I said.

She peered into my eyes for a second, drew her hand back and walked ahead of me. I had pulled the wrong card again. Better stay mum the rest of the way, I thought, reaching for my bag to get the umbrella.

'Hey!' she called me from the other side of the road. 'Do you need that now? The rain has stopped, I guess.'

The rain gods heard that and didn't like it. And so the rain returned with a bang. I rushed towards her with my umbrella but she seemed to be lost in her own world. She was enjoying the feel of the rain on her outstretched arms and stood looking up at the sky. She closed her eyes as the heavy raindrops kissed her face. I didn't disturb her; I stood watching from a distance because it was so amazing to watch her madness under those dim street lights. If the rain was at its best, would the wind be far behind? It too came down roaring, even more fiercely this time, and blew away my umbrella. I ran behind it but she stopped me, grabbing my arms.

'Let it go, we don't need it.'

'It's raining,' I said, but I dissented.

'It would be harsh if I used your umbrella, leaving you in the rain.'

'What?' I grimaced.

'Well, I guess you're too gentlemanly to let a woman get drenched nor would I do that to you, and no way am I coming with you in the same umbrella,' she said with a naughty smile on her face. She was still holding my arms.

If not the rain, her touch gave me shivers. I left the umbrella behind and walked with her to the station, which was some two miles from the pub. They say such a moment comes along once in everyone's life, but I never thought it would come to us so early. I don't mean early in our 'relationship', because we weren't a couple yet. So what had brought her so close to me, I never quite understood. She was clinging to my shoulders now. I could feel the warmth of her breath on my drenched skin and it gave me goosebumps. Gosh! It was one of those moments when you begin to understand Einstein's Theory of Relativity. Seriously, was it two miles or two steps?

I'd always admired women in saris; even if otherwise not beautiful, a sari made a woman definitely look sexy. But the rain had made Ananya absolutely aphrodisiacal. And I wasn't her only admirer there at the station. It was around eleven, we were waiting for the last train to Panvel. Thane station wasn't too crowded, just a handful of commuters, a few urchins and stray loafers idling around. They occasionally stole glances at her and taunted us from a distance. But she didn't seem to mind. Perhaps, she took their glances as a compliment. And as if that weren't enough, two little kids tugged at our clothes, asking for money, knowing well that couples are always a soft target. When we didn't budge though, they gave up. Last came an elderly fat lady who made me get up from the bench because it was meant for ladies, though it would easily have accommodated two more like her, besides me and Ananya. She gave me such a dirty look seeing my reluctance, one would think I was sitting with her daughter. I felt very awkward, standing there like a fool while Ananya sat glued to my iPad. Motion sensor games I tell you!

Lucky for me that the rain hadn't delayed the trains. I saw the bright headlight far across the tracks, followed by the loud whistle echoing through the empty station. Ananya was too engrossed in the game to realize that the train had arrived, I pulled her by her hand and the old lady almost raised an alarm seeing this. I instantly dropped Ananya's hand in terror and moved ahead. But it didn't take Ananya even a fraction of a second to get a hold of the situation; she stuck to my side and clasped my fingers in hers, tightly. A shock of a thousand volts ran down my veins but she just winked at me. I could see the confused defeat on the face of that woman as we boarded the train; I wanted to see her expression till the train moved away, so we stood at the door still hand in hand.

As the train moved, Ananya stood right at the edge of the footboard and leaned outside, holding the bar, to feel the breeze. The train hadn't yet moved out of the station completely, the loafers were still there, and as they noticed her, they screamed all sorts of lewd comments and began item chants. She wasn't bothered one bit but of course, it hurt me, badly. The bloody male ego again! I pushed her in and asked her to go sit down.

'What's wrong now?' she shrugged off my hand. My grip had actually left a bruise around her arm.

'Didn't you see that?'

'What should I see? If they are shouting what can I do?'

'See, I don't want to fight with you here. Just go in and sit there.'

'Who the hell are you to order me like that? Are you my boyfriend or something?' she railed.

I shook my head and stayed mum. She leaned against the wall and looked out. I kept staring at her, hoping for our eyes to meet, but she just ignored me.

'Ananya,' I called out but she didn't turn around. 'Damn! Don't you see how much I care for you?'

'That's my question, why do you care?' she was fuming. I didn't have an answer. She waved me aside and went in to take a seat. I didn't follow her, I stayed at the door, holding the bar and the door clamp, and turned to look out.

Ours wasn't a perfect friendship, free from problems and misunderstandings. Perhaps, it was one in which a sorry and a smile always made everything perfect as before, but then it never got intense. I used to feel bad about that. But did it bother her one bit? Nah, she was always busy with her SMSs. I too gave up the thought of persuading her.

The train had crossed half the distance when it began to drizzle again. I still hung on to the door, but a few minutes later, I realized it was a bad idea. I didn't love the rain like she did. I looked inside but I was still upset. I looked at her; she had slipped her hand out of the window and was playing with the drops dripping in through the window pane. *And she says she is twenty-eight*, I thought to myself.

'Gautam,' she called, 'come inside and sit.'

'I'm fine,' I said curtly. I wanted her to know how hurt I still was.

'OK, as you wish,' she went back to flirting with the rain.

The rain had picked up, I had closed the door but it didn't help at all. A stream of water gushed in from the roof of the train, soaking me fully, again. I still didn't move from the door area; I wanted to know how long she would ignore my pain. But she didn't look at me even once. I gave up after some time and sat on the seat opposite her. I didn't talk to her though.

'Finally!' She sprinkled some water in my direction. I returned a dirty look but her naughty smile yet again mended all woes between us.

'I'm sorry for everything,' I said. 'I just…'

'Stop!' she interrupted me, 'Don't start it all over again. Let's talk something else.'

Between us, she always did most of the talking. She had once said that my stories were boring; also, she assumed that I loved listening to her. Sometimes, I would just stare into those dazzling kohl-lined eyes or simply play with her nails which always had some sort of art on them. She would tell me one story after another and I would react as her eyes demanded, I could read them. I wished these moments could last a lifetime, but then, Mumbai locals are too quick.

'Well, just one stop to go,' I grimaced, as the train crossed Khandeshwar.

'Hmmm.' She gave a long sigh.

'Can I drop you home?' I asked her sheepishly.

'No, Gautam, I can go alone.'

'But it's too late!' I tried to argue.

'I said no,' she said sternly.

Silence.

'Would you tell me something honestly?' she asked. I nodded.

'Do you love me?'

Long silence.

She was twenty-eight.

She had a psycho boyfriend for four years.

She was to get married in a few months.

And I loved Riya.

I couldn't utter a word in reply. I wondered what made her feel like asking that question. I glanced at her, but she wasn't looking at me. Her eyes reflected guilt. That bolt-from-the-blue question had actually crossed an invisible boundary line between us. It had messed things up, I knew at once. The word 'love' is *that* offensive. We stayed quiet the rest of the time, careful not to let our eyes meet.

'Good night,' she said, as she got off the train. I nodded and followed her silently.

The world always seemed to come to an end every time she walked away, but I would wait and watch her go, until she crossed the bridge. She usually never turned back. But that night she did. If not her words, at least her eyes still demanded a reply.

Those unsaid words were smothering me. She had reached halfway on the bridge; a few more seconds of standing there and I would have let her go. I would see her again the next day, I said to myself. But that period in between, it seemed to last forever. It was the last train for the day waiting on the platform, but I couldn't wait until morning. A phone call or an SMS was not an option anymore. I wanted to tell her right then. I didn't want her to leave.

'Ananya,' I shouted, as I reached the bridge. She was near the parking area. She looked back at me; she knew what I was up to. She shook her head. I could see the pain in her eyes. She didn't want a scene again, nor did I. I ran down the bridge to reach her as fast as I could and when I reached there, she wasn't waiting.

She was gone.

I'm Broke-up, Love Me

Six months before I met Ananya...

The first thing I did as I lifted my head from the pillow was to check my cell phone. There was still no sign of her. I called her, she didn't pick up again. I checked the time, it was already 11. *What was wrong? Was she fine?* I worried, as usual. However, I was feeling too lazy to get up and go to her house. I had slept very late last night. It was actually my birthday and she had never missed being the first to wish me. But yesterday, she hadn't called me at all, and while waiting for her, I ended up attending all the calls and replying to all the SMSs I got. I called her on her cell phone a couple of times and also sent her a few messages but she didn't respond. Finally, I dialled her landline at home but immediately disconnected, realizing it was too late. Her behaviour was a bit strange over the last few days, and I was feeling restless thinking about what was possibly going on between us.

I logged on to Facebook and checked her profile. Her status had read 'In a relationship with Gautam Deshmukh' since the day she had joined Facebook. Now it was gone, she had changed it to 'Single'. On the left, below her display picture, her number of photos was reduced to about fifteen from more than the two hundred there had been before. She had not only removed most of the photos from her albums but had also untagged herself from other's photos. I didn't understand what was she up to.

'Riya!' She had finally picked up my call in the morning.

'Hi, Gautam! Happy birthday!' she wished me, but something was missing. Her love.

'I thought you forgot it.'

'No way, how could I?'

'You didn't call me last night. I was waiting for your call. You always wished me…'

'I'm sorry. I slept early yesterday,' she said coldly.

'It's OK, sweetheart. I don't mind that. Our love is not bound by all this…'

'What's the plan for tonight?' she interrupted me again.

'Oh, a big bash, close friends and my sweetheart.'

'No. Let's celebrate the occasion with just you and me, no one else.'

'As you wish, Sweetie.'

'OK, see you then in the evening. Bye,' she hung up.

∽

She was already waiting for me at the gate of her building. *She didn't want me to come up to her house?* That was indeed a stupid thought; I pushed it out of my mind. Her parents never had any problems with me. Sometimes, they gave me company when Riya kept me waiting; she took ages to get ready. But the way she wore her earrings (she had a huge collection to choose from), gently lined her almond eyes (probably the most beautiful eyes I have ever seen), pressed her lips close to make her lip-gloss spread out evenly (I didn't even recognize some of the colours she had) always fascinated me, but I'd never told her about it. Once done, she would step away from her dressing table and strike a pose; I would just flash her a big smile. No matter how breathtakingly beautiful she looked, I never complimented her.

She was wearing a pale blue kurta and jeans without a hint of make-up; I realized that's how she had made it on time. She still looked stunning, her long streaked hair blew with the breeze and covered her melancholic beautiful face, but she didn't try to move the strands away from her face. She stood calm and still. She was lost somewhere; actually she wasn't the Riya I had known for so long. Something was definitely wrong.

'Hi Sweetie!' I said. She grinned, pressing her lips together.

'Where to?' she asked as she got in the car. Strange! She had never asked me that before. I would just hold her hand and she would walk with me without asking me where and why.

'It's a surprise, Babe!' I smiled.

There was an uncomfortable silence between us inside the car. She wasn't talking to me, wasn't fighting with me over the music and wasn't teasing me for putting on weight either. She was quiet, looking outside the window. I too didn't try anything to change her mood. I wanted to surprise her. If things were really not going well between us, I knew exactly how to cheer her up. It was time to show her what she meant to me and to say to her all those unsaid words that I had stored away somewhere in my mind for the right occasion. And this was it!

I drove ahead of our school towards the hills and as I took the turn to climb to the top, she sensed what was coming. I should have asked her to close her eyes, stupid me! But I thought the excitement was enough to get her going. However, she remained cold. I saw a little smile on her face yet it was nothing compared to what I expected. I mean, this was the very place where I had confessed my love to her some years ago. I don't really remember the exact date; it was the annual day of her school. She had asked me to come and see her dance but I had preferred playing snooker with my friends at City Mall.

∽

'Dude! I swear I saw her with him many times. They go to the same tutor. You see the school, then the class and later the walk, don't you think it's a bit too much?' Pradeep was talking about some guy whom he believed Riya was probably seeing.

I ignored him and concentrated on my game.

'I also heard that he is her dance partner for tonight's performance,' he continued.

'So?' I snapped.

'Don't you care for the fact? Aren't you jealous? Don't you love her?'

'Dude! Just stop,' I interrupted him even as his expressions still demanded answers. 'Well, we have been together as long as I remember and I do like her very much.'

'Have you told her?'

I shook my head.

'Well, then I suggest you tell her before it gets too late.'

Ex-students are treated well in our school; I got a seat in the front row. However, only a few of the teachers' pets had turned up for the programme. Needless to say, I was damn bored in the company of those geeks, I thought I'd send Riya a message saying that I had come, and then I'd leave. But then, after seeing some of the performances, I felt that it wasn't that bad after all. When I was a kid, I too used to participate in a lot of such events and my parents never missed any of them. Regardless of how bad I was on stage, they always appreciated me. But later, as a teenager, I found these things embarrassing and I kept myself away from it all. So, this was like revisiting my childhood days. I smiled recalling those innocent memories and put my phone back in my pocket. I decided to watch the entire programme.

I never felt as excited as I did that day, hearing her name as the anchor announced her performance. She came onstage with her group. She was wearing a long Cinderella dress and behind her glasses, I knew her eyes were searching for me. I waved at her from my seat, she immediately turned away, but then the smile on her face was just for me. It was a Salsa dance set to the romantic *Tumse se hi* song from *Jab We Met* and as it started, I realized that Pradeep had been right about everything. That guy was her partner, and each time he picked her up or even held her hand, I almost skipped a heartbeat. I did care. I was jealous indeed. Was I really in love with Riya?

I didn't wait a second after the performance was over; I went to see her backstage. She was there with her dance troop. They shouted, they danced and congratulated each other. They had won the first prize and were high on the celebrations. I made my way through the bizarre sets and looked for Riya. She was with a couple of girls, standing on a platform, posing for photographs. I waited to the side for her to finish but she saw me.

'Hey! Thanks for coming,' she came up to me and smiled.

'My pleasure,' I beamed. 'You look so pretty today.'

'Thank you,' she blushed.

'Can we just go out a bit? I want to tell you something,' I said apprehensively. She looked into my eyes; there was something different about that stare, as if she had known what I was up to. But what was on her mind? I just couldn't read it, but at least, I saw a bit of affection for me in those haunting eyes.

'Hey!' the same guy piped in, 'Riya! Can I have a photo of yours?'

'Sure,' she shrugged.

'Dude! Would you move aside a bit? You are coming within the frame,' he said to me. This annoyed me, more so because he was by then standing right next to her and I had to move aside for them both. He clicked a photo of her alone and ran up to her to show her the picture. She blushed as he praised her, and I felt the heat rising in me. I wanted to hit him hard.

'Hey! Can you just click one photo of us, together?' It was meant to be a request, but the way he said it, it sounded like a lot more; especially the last word 'together' echoed in my mind like my morning alarm. I glared at him furiously but he didn't care; instead, gave me his camera to click a picture. Of course, the first thing that crossed my mind was to smash the camera into pieces but the gadget was too good to be destroyed. I have a great respect for brands, you see. And as I clicked their photo, he snatched the camera almost instantly after the flash and retrieved the photo to show it to her. What followed was some more admiration, praises and giggles, with the two of them standing close. Too close. I was not angry or jealous anymore; I was hurt. I felt as if a fire was lit beneath my heart. I wanted to hurt that jerk by slowly twisting out his finger nails one by one. I wanted her to know that I was feeling left out and hurt but she was too caught up in the merrymaking. And that just did it for me. I stormed out of the place in anguish.

'Gautam!' somebody called. I turned around. Riya had followed me to the parking lot. I only stopped when I was near my bike; she almost jogged the remaining distance.

'Hey! What's wrong?' she was panting.

'What?' I tried being indifferent.

'Why did you leave?'

'It's too late. I need to go home.'

'Really?' she smirked. 'Does Gautam Deshmukh care about time?'

'Whatever? I am leaving,' and I mounted my bike.

'That's so rude! Anyway, I need a lift back home,' she didn't wait for my nod; she was already astride, sitting pillion, before she finished her sentence.

We had just gone a few metres when I felt her hands over my shoulders, and after a little bump on a speed breaker, she held me even tighter. This wasn't exactly the first time that I was giving her a ride, and yet I wondered whether she had always put her arms around me that way. Maybe I had never noticed it earlier, and if so, then I had been such a dork to ignore it till date. We had known each other and had spent time together all life! And that's what had actually cemented our feelings for each other over time, yet it required a geek like Pradeep to make us realize it. But then, I didn't want to wait any longer to express my mind to her.

Yeah! Gautam Deshmukh really doesn't care about the time, I muttered and turned my bike off the main road, towards the hills. She asked me about where we were heading but I chose not to answer her, and she didn't ask me again either. I guess she had sensed my instincts, but she wasn't protesting. Moreover, her heavy breath on the back of my neck gave me goosebumps and made the blood rush in my veins.

I stopped as we reached the peak and by the time I put my bike on the stand and locked it, she had walked right till the edge. It just seemed perfect to go after her and take her in my arms, but I hadn't made her mine yet, so I stood beside her instead. Our hands entwined, she looked at me and smiled. At that very moment, I felt like kissing her and telling her how much I loved her. But love is not that easy to confess, so both of us remained mum, either measuring the ends of the city stretched out in front of us or simply counting the stars.

'I think we should leave now,' she checked the time on her cell phone, it was near midnight.

'Wait, I've got something to tell you,' I mumbled, and she looked at me eagerly. That thing called love was actually bringing out all the stupid nervousness in me, as I stood before her, phrasing the words in my mind, and I could see excitement in her eyes, seeing how nervous I had grown.

'Gautam, be quick, it's getting late,' she said.

'Well…is it really necessary that I should say it?' I struggled with my words; her eyes still wanted me to confess it, I could see. 'I mean you already know what I want to say.'

'Like what?' she was exasperated.

'C'mon, you know it.'

'No. I don't,' she turned away and walked towards the bike.

'What? Wait! Let me finish,' I ran after her but she didn't stop.

'Damn! I wanted to say that I love you,' the words rushed out of my mouth and I stood aghast. She turned to face me immediately.

'What did you say?' she had a slick smile on her face.

'You already heard it and now you answer,' I said.

'But I guess that wasn't a question, it was just a statement about what you feel for me,' she giggled. 'So how could you expect an answer from me?'

I was never a charmer, but if you really wish to date a girl like Riya, the expectations are a lot higher. Maybe I needed to write her name on the moon or simply hire Enrique to sing my feelings to her. Whatever. That was just the best effort I could do at that moment and I knew I was nowhere near impressing her. I hung my head sheepishly.

'No wonder, you still remain a dork,' she reached for me, put her arms around my shoulder, around my neck and pulled me closer. I wanted to look into her eyes to know what they wanted but they were already closed, she wanted me to kiss her.

That was our first kiss. Was it good or bad? We didn't know, we had nothing to compare it with. It wasn't about the lips fighting to dominate or a sloppy exchange of saliva or the tongue exploring it all. Though it did happen that way, but it's hard to explain the experience in mere words. There was nothing logical about it; it just gave us this beautiful feeling of belonging, the feeling of being loved by someone, and it made us forget everything around us and we never wanted it to come to an end. And when it did end, I found my hands around her waist and her fingers had messed up my hair. We smiled, looking into each other's eyes, and we kissed again.

∽

After so many years of togetherness, we were back at the same place where it had all begun. Strange though! It was just our second visit after that night, yet nothing seemed to have changed much, only this time it was a Beetle instead of a CBZ. I stopped the car and put on some light jazz music. Her favourite. And the music did the trick, she turned to me. She was smiling, finally. She put her hand over mine; her touch still sent a current through my body. I clasped her fingers in mine and reached for her. Her eyes neither seemed romantic nor naughty, I still kissed her. But then there was something missing; it didn't feel right somehow, her affection for me and our love wasn't the same anymore. She wasn't mine anymore. I pushed her back. She didn't dare to look at me.

'What's wrong with you?' I yelled at her. She looked down. I lifted her face with my palm under her chin; she had tears in her eyes. I got my answer.

'You want to break-up with me?'

She didn't reply, she just softly wept. I waited for her to stop.

'Is there any other guy?' I asked. She shook her head. I asked her again, raising my voice this time.

'You know Gautam, how much I love you,' she said and looked down. If not fear, her voice had a trace of guilt in it.

'Then?'

'I just don't want it.'

'What?'

'This relationship,' she said finally, looking at me.

It took me some time to digest those words. She was still crying, tears rolling down her cheeks. It hurt her too. Then why? What had gone wrong? Gawking at her, red faced, I clutched the steering wheel hard and sat listening to her low sobs. I felt a big lump in my throat impelling me to cry too. It took an effort of a lifetime to remain calm.

'Thanks! For this lovely birthday gift.'

'See, it isn't your fault,' she said in a choked voice. I still didn't react. Perhaps, I actually didn't want to know. The reason might hurt even more, I thought.

'I'm going to the US to do research,' she continued.

'So?'

'I don't want to carry this relationship there. I don't want to miss you there.'

'What do you mean by that? Won't you come back here?'

She shook her head. 'I don't know what's there for me in the future nor do I want to think about it. I just want to concentrate on my career. And I don't want anything back there which would divert my mind. See, distant relationships don't work anyway,' her justifications just weren't strong enough to convince me. I glared at her angrily.

'Is your research that important to you?'

'Yes, it is. I don't have a rich dad like you do. I need to do something of my own.'

'What's this something of your own?' I demanded.

'I'm fed up of being in your shadow. I just need a bit of independence. I don't want you to boss my life anymore. I need to breathe free.'

'It's been seven years. Damn! How can you be so mean? Don't you care about me? About us?'

'Us? There wasn't anything like that. It was always about you and your family.'

'Mind your words, Riya. Don't dare to drag in my family here,' I shouted.

'Really?' She sighed. 'Let's face it, Gautam. You're talking about seven years, why go that far? Just look back at the last two years of your life. Since you graduated, have you done anything for yourself? You're just nothing without your dad's name.'

'What?' I reacted instantly in dismay. 'Damn! I stood third in the university papers and my final year project on a computer interface which tracks eye movements won awards at international forums. I was a boxing champ at college level. And those quiz competitions, debates and all; have you forgotten? I was the student of the year for four consecutive years in school.'

'So? Life isn't about grades, medals and work outs. Have you ever thought of getting a job and earning some money of your own?'

'Why should I go for a job? I've got a big business to handle,' I defended.

'Oh really? Tell me, how many times you have been to your office in these two years? And anyway, if you were to handle a business then why did you do engineering?'

'Because Dad wanted me to do it.'

'And you did what he said. That's my point; you do whatever your Dad says to you. He wanted you to leave boxing, you left. He wanted you to do engineering, you did. He wanted you to stay back and you didn't join any company. He wants you to do nothing and enjoy life, you're doing that. He's been controlling everything in your life and you never protest. At the end, he has just ruined you because at twenty-four, even after being so bright, you're just a bloody loser.'

'Just shut up,' I screamed at her.

'Stop it now. If you want to go, you go. I won't stop you.' And that actually stopped her for a moment.

'If your Dad wants, you would even leave me na?'

'It's not about him. It's you who's leaving,' I blinked back the tears in my eyes, but she didn't care, she turned away to look out of the car window.

For the rest of the ride back home, we didn't talk to each other. She sat staring outside the window. I glanced at her, I could see her reflection in the glass; she was still crying. Her presence was actually killing my insides, and I drove in full speed. I just couldn't tolerate her anymore. She warned me a few times, but I didn't pay any heed, all I wanted was for her to be out of my car, out of my sight and out of my life.

She took an eternity to get off as I stopped at her building gate. She bid me goodbye and gave a peck on my cheeks, I shrugged and looked away in the opposite direction. She was standing outside my car and I rudely shut the door close without saying a word. I stepped hard on the accelerator and was off. A few metres away, I glanced at my rearview mirror. She was still standing there as she always did, watching me go.

I got home and silently walked in the door without anybody noticing; a debate on my break-up with Riya was the last thing I wanted on my birthday. I slipped into my room and locked the door. I flopped down on the bed thinking of everything that happened. I still couldn't believe that she had broken up with me; I checked my cell phone haplessly for her message or call. She always called, just to know whether I had reached home safely. But that day, there wasn't anything like that. My ego was preventing me from calling her, but my love for her had made me weak, and I dialled her number.

'Riya!' I yelled at her.

'You reached home?' her concern gave me solace. *She still cared, she still loved me. It wasn't over yet.*

'Yes, baby!' I gasped, 'I love you Riya.'

'Gautam, please! Don't make things difficult for me. Don't call me or message me again.'

'Don't say like that please…' but before I could complete my sentence, she had cut the call.

I tried her number again; after ringing for a few times, it stopped. I tried again, it was not reachable. I messaged her but I didn't receive any delivery report. It was over, she was gone. I threw my phone on the floor in frustration, it broke into pieces, and so did my heart. I don't know why they call it just heartbreak. It felt like every other part of my body was broken too. Images of her kept hovering in my head only to make me realize what she meant to me. I sat huddled on the bed, holding my knees tightly drawn up to my chest. And I cried.

DevD Syndrome

Time went by, life moved on, but all I could think of was why she was gone. Why did those feelings have to be so true? Why did I care so deeply about her? I wished I could just forget about her like she had forgotten about me. I felt restless as thoughts of her kept bothering me.

I was waiting for Sahil by the roadside. I couldn't stand around idle. So I lit a cigarette out of habit, to kill all feeling. I had to do something, anything, to keep myself from thinking about her. Smoking was one of the many ways I had found of avoiding reality and not facing myself, of not giving in to the fight between me and my conscience. But instead of offering any comfort or peace of mind, smoking had actually made me realize how much I hated myself. By the time Sahil came along, I had smoked about five cigarettes. The way I saw it, it made my lungs black and I wanted something that would burn my heart.

'Hey!' Sahil gave me a high-five as he stopped his bike.

'So, what's the plan for today?' I asked.

'Sinhagad fort.'

'Aah...' I moaned.

'What's wrong with you these days?'

'Actually, I don't want to be with these people anymore.'

'Why?'

'You know the reason.'

'What?'

'This is the reason,' I showed him the dark spot near my elbow. 'Mom saw it the other day and has been nagging about this ever since.'

'I understand.'

'See, smoking and boozing is OK but not drugs and all. I think we still have time to get over this, the situation has not worsened that much yet.'

'You want to move out?' he asked and I hung my head. 'Listen dude! You weren't forced to join us, you only came to us. And I guess you don't want your dad to know about your late night adventures,' he threatened. He had a point blank expression on his face, I could see he meant the warning. He had hit the right nerve; I had no choice other than to accompany him.

∽

After Riya left me, my life seemed to have regressed. I felt completely shattered. For the first few days, I stayed locked up in my room; I didn't talk to anybody about it, I just cried all day, thinking about her. I dialled her number repeatedly, only to realize that she had changed it. My calls never reached her; she had blocked me on all chat messengers. I couldn't even see her wall posts on Facebook, she had 'un-friended' me. She had completely deleted me from her life.

The pain was so bad, I felt that had my heart stopped beating, it wouldn't have hurt as much. With every passing day it grew worse, until one day, I stepped out of my home in search of solace, and ended up exploring the dark streets of the city. The DevD syndrome, as they call it, took over, and I spent my nights in either pubs or parties. I drank more alcohol than water, and I didn't breathe, I only smoked. I injected drugs and made friends who had criminal records. In a way, I was running away from my life.

On one of those crazy nights, I met them—Michael, Sahil and Raghu. They claimed to be BPO professionals but that seemed contrary to the fact that they owned a plush apartment in the heart of the city and drove a Honda Civic! Actually, they dealt in drugs, and if rumours were to be believed, they had links with the mafia. I had also seen Michael carrying a pistol with him. The police were on a hunt for him for some time now, which was thwarting their habits and they badly needed me to fund them. I had known about this from the start, yet I never tried hard enough to move out, maybe because I had my own needs. I needed them to save me from the emptiness in my life. I needed them to surround me with madness to help me forget Riya. I needed them for the drugs to prevent the hole in my heart from bleeding.

But I couldn't go any further with them; I had to part ways, not because I was done destroying myself, but to guard my name. Moreover, I feared Dad, not because he would hate me but because he loved me too much. So, that was to be my last outing with them; I decided to talk to Michael and explain that I wanted to return home.

'Whatever. I'll talk to them about it,' I said aloud boldly, as we sat on Sahil's bike.

'Your call, but I guess it's better for you not to spoil Michael's mood on his birthday.'

Sahil drove into the jungle just behind the fort corridor. It was pitch dark and the silence would have given anyone a good shiver. As we made our way further in, I could hear rock music and see a campfire in the distance. The party was on in full swing. As we reached the spot, I could see many youngsters had gathered. A few foreigners, students from nearby colleges and some locals; about thirty people in all. It was a gathering for the dopers in the city, organized by Michael.

Brown sugar, heroin, cocaine—all these I had just heard about before in Bollywood movies of the seventies, where villains smuggled them in through the sea. There was a heap of cigarette boxes, syringes, drug packets, and everything else that seemed contraband. Some people injected, some licked, some filled in their cigarettes and smoked them, and some others sucked in the dope directly through the nose. They rolled, they shouted, they sang and they danced. I definitely didn't belong there.

'Hi Bro! You're so late for my birthday,' Michael greeted. It didn't matter whether it was a birthday or an anniversary; life itself was a big party for Michael.

'Happy birthday,' I wished him coldly.

'Hey! Where is my gift?' he demanded like a child.

'What do you want?' I was trying not to be rude.

'I just want to see a little smile on my brother's face.'

I gave him a small smile. He gave me a hug.

'Michael, I need to talk.'

'Now?'

'Yep.'

'What?' He had sensed what was to come.

'See...I want to get out of here,' I approached tentatively.

'Sure. Go home. After the party,' he snubbed.

'I won't tell anybody.'

'What would you not tell anyone?' he violently shoved me towards a tree trunk and held me by my collar, others rushed in to separate us.

'I mean it, I'm leaving,' I growled, as Raghu and Sahil pulled him away from me. The party had stopped.

Michael didn't like rebels around him and my tone had made my meaning perfectly clear. He pushed both of his sidekicks aside and pounced at me. I was still on the ground, getting my bearings, when he kicked me. Once. Twice. Thrice. I groaned in pain and he thought it was over for sure. But I was adamant and told him again that I wanted to move out. Sahil helped me to get back on my feet while I kept staring at Michael furiously.

'What the hell are you looking at? You bloody son of a bitch,' he howled.

'Just mind your language.' My temper was building up.

'What did you say?' he was back again, pushing me backward with his forceful jabs.

'Don't dare to do anything now,' I warned. He didn't know that I had had a lot of practice at boxing since the age of twelve. He pumped his fist and hurled a punch at me, I craned my neck backward and he missed. Before he could even blink, I shocked him with a powerful cross punch, delivered straight at his nose. It broke and began bleeding.

'Fuck!' he cried, 'Someone hold him!'

His men rushed at me. I tried to run but they grabbed me. I kicked, punched and did a lot to break free, but my efforts were in vain. They soon took control of me. Michael filled a syringe, I don't know with what, but I was sure that it wasn't some vitamin. I struggled even harder but ten men are enough to tame even Arnold. He injected the syringe into my arm, and in the next moment, I felt my senses block up immediately. I couldn't get a hold on any part of my body, forget about standing on my feet. I felt as if I didn't have any bones inside my body, the world around me was spinning very fast and my head was pounding. After that I think they beat me black and blue.

I didn't know what they really wanted to do with me. I must have been unconscious for a while, and I was woken by the hustle of many people around me. The police were here! They shouted out orders and ran in all directions. I didn't want to get caught in the police raid. I tried to stand but couldn't. So then I tried to crawl my way to safety, and after a few yards, I rolled downhill. The last thing I remember was hearing the sound of bullets. I never figured out how I made my way to the highway and then home.

∽

'Gautam, wake up! It's almost eleven!' Mom was calling out for the third time.

I was at home, in my room, on my bed. My first thought was, *nothing happened last night, I just had a nightmare*. I tried to get up but instantly realized that everything hurt. My back was stiff, my neck ached, and when I finally managed to sit up, a stabbing pain coursed through my shoulder.

'Where were you last night? Your shoes are full of mud,' Mom said, looking at the footprints all over the floor.

So it wasn't a dream, I grimaced as I looked in the mirror. The scars on my face were evidence of everything that had happened in the night. I was quick to rush to the bathroom to avoid Mom's questions. I looked at myself in the mirror, leaning on the basin. My legs were trembling, tears rolled down my cheeks and a strange spasm of pain coming from my chest racked my whole body, as I recalled the events of the night.

'Gautam! Come outside, somebody has come for you,' Didi knocked at the door.

'Who?' I sneaked out.

'Don't know. Mom just told me to call you.'

I reckoned what was in store for me. My sins were too big to overlook. Those few minutes of introspection under the shower had given me some strength. I was ready to face the consequences. But as I saw the police officer talking with Dad, I felt the adrenaline rush through my body, my heart thump, and my feet felt like they were made of lead. A voice within was persuading me to run but the guilt held me back. I tried my best to appear normal but the forced and fake smile on my face was not good enough.

'Hello,' the officer greeted me.

'Hi!'

'Do you know him?' he showed me a photo of Michael.

'Yes…but not closely,' I said, looking at Dad. It was not that easy to get away from the situation.

'Really? But his phone records said he called you regularly,' he retorted firmly, looking me straight in the eye, and my blood froze in fear.

'He is just a casual friend,' I defended.

'He was killed last night in an encounter.'

'Oh, I don't know anything,' I broke down.

'Really? Where were you last night?'

'Officer, you are crossing your limits,' Dad interrupted, seeing me uncomfortable.

'It's a part of the investigation,' the officer persisted.

'I was at Lions Club,' I piped in.

'OK now tell me, what happened to your mouth?' He had noticed the cut on my lips.

'I told you I was in the club. I was practicing boxing. I got this from there.'

'The other guy named Sahil who is in our custody has taken your name and we also found your cell phone with him,' so saying, he showed me my phone. *Sahil had always been tempted to flick my phone*, I thought. Damn!

'Well…' the interrogation was getting worse. 'I don't know how but I lost it last night in the club.'

'I guess that's enough for now. You may leave,' Dad intervened again. The inspector's phone began ringing shrilly; Dad had called a few people, I assumed. From the inspector's expression, I guessed he had been asked to drop the interrogation and leave immediately, probably by his senior and probably with some choice words thrown in.

'OK fine. I'll leave but it's not over yet,' he looked baffled and stormed away.

Dad didn't say anything but his eyes demanded an explanation.

'I don't know any of it,' I defended.

He smiled and patted my back, 'I know beta.'

Over the next few days, due to media hype, Sahil's case was gathering momentum. His involvement with the drugs had only added fuel to the fire and was actually making things worse for me. Dad had used all his contacts to protect me, but when I saw the reports constantly being aired on news channels, I knew the day wasn't far when the police would put the handcuffs on me. Dad didn't ask me anything about that night though, nor did anyone else in my home speak about it. It only meant two possibilities; either they had sensed the truth or they just trusted me that much. In either case, I had killed their trust. Days passed and there was an uncomfortable silence building between me and my family. I avoided them as much as possible, seeing them only at dinner; all other times, I remained inside my room, cursing myself in despair. Sometimes, I did feel like confessing, but then I would wonder how to explain that it wasn't exactly my fault, and I would change my mind. However, each day my pain only grew more intense, and locking myself in the room was no remedy. I thought about moving into a new place, at least till the matter was settled. No more bad ways, no more punishing myself. I wanted to live a new, improved life.

'Dad!' I had decided to talk to him.

'Yes?'

'I want to tell you something…I…want to do something with my life.'

'That's great. You can join our office. I will find something for you to do there.'

'No Dad. I don't want your help. I will do something by myself.'

'What exactly?'

'A job in some company. I mean, I am an engineer after all,' I said.

'Are you serious?' Dad was surprised.

I nodded. 'I will take up a job in Mumbai or some other city.'

'What? Why not this city? Pune has a lot of scope in the IT field. I will talk to somebody.'

'No Dad. Don't do that. I want a big change in my life. I need to be independent. I want to start from zero,' I explained. That didn't go down well with him; he gave me a cold stare and then turned away.

'I'm sorry Dad. I don't want to be in your shadow anymore.'

Silence.

'Beta,' he turned to me again and smiled. 'I knew this was coming.'

'What?!'

'Why do you think I asked you to stop boxing or didn't allow you to go abroad?'

I shook my head.

'See, whatever I have, it's all yours. I always had this fear. What if you ignore all this and go away to do something on your own. Whatever you do in your life, you simply go beyond everything. What would have happened if I had allowed you to take up boxing seriously, you might have gone to the Olympics! Or if you were allowed to go abroad, who knows whether you would have done something great there and never returned? And then what about all this? Who would have run this empire after me? So, in a way I let you run carefree so that you never leave us.'

His words actually freaked me out and I began thinking about whether I would really be able to survive outside alone. I was thoroughly confused.

'Dad! I still insist. Maybe just a few years, say two. Let me explore the outside world.'

Dad smiled a lot that day, a strange smile. 'I know son, you won't return, and I think I should not stop you either. It's your life after all. You may go. All the best.'

I hugged him tight.

Like in the Movies

A month after I came to Mumbai.

My phone beeped. 'Let's move.'

I glanced at the right corner of my screen, it was already 5.57. Three minutes to go, I was late! I jumped off my seat, pulled out the mobile charger, unwound my headphones, grabbed all the stuff on my desk and threw them into my bag. Two minutes left! Hell, I didn't even have time to shut down the machine properly. I glanced around, nobody was looking; I simply leaned behind my monitor, switched off my system and began to run.

'Deshmukh!' *Panauti* called out.

'Yes Sir!' I turned to face him with a tight smile.

'Where are you going?' he asked.

'Well…home, Sir.' My fake smile turned into a sheepish grin.

'So early?' he snapped. His gaze wiped away my smile and I looked at my feet. 'I want that Network report.'

'Now?!' I asked.

'I guess that's not a question!' He had the most cunning smile on his face.

I went back to my seat, cursing myself for switching off the system. These childish morals I had—save power, save the earth and whatnot. *Goddamn! I need to grow up*, I mumbled to myself as I thumped my bag on the desk. I flicked the switch on and parked my butt in the chair. The computer booted and a couple of seconds later, it was asking whether I wanted to scan my disk because of the improper shutdown. I had ten seconds to think but my fingers had already reached the spacebar.

'Hey! Stop!' Muthu screamed in my ears and I withdrew my hands in shock.

Time's up.

C:\ scanning...

'What?' I reacted.

'Let the CPU do the scanning, it's important,' he directed. *Fuck you asshole!* I didn't have to say that, my expression said it all.

I waited another five minutes to hear the Windows musical as my system completed the check. Life was really tough, what with those primitive machines. The clock showed 6.07, I checked my cell phone. Three missed calls and two messages, all from Ananya.

Message 1: *Whr r u?*

Message 2: *Pick ma cal.*

I replied: *M late ☹ will meet u directly @ station.*

'Keep that phone down and send the mail.' Muthu was still hovering over my head.

I put my phone down. 'Outlook is opening, Sir,' I said, and browsed through my drives for the document. When the going is tough, it gets tougher! I kept double clicking on folder after folder to locate the file; I had forgotten where I had saved it. Finally, I keyed in the file name in the Search bar, knowing this would only take more time. I scrolled through all the file names as the little pup on the screen kept turning pages.

'Who's this Ananya?' Muthu asked and I looked at him perplexed.

Damn! My phone was in his hand and he was scrolling through my message inbox! I snatched my phone back instantly. 'Sir, that's personal.'

He didn't react, just beamed at me. I returned to my screen, disgusted.

'Is she your girlfriend?' he continued irritating me but I didn't bother to reply; I had found the file and was uploading it as an attachment.

'OK, don't reply, but make sure you use the right fonts for the report.'

'Done!' I said as I clicked on the Send button.

'OK! Wait till I review it,' he said, still smiling, and I was so tempted to give his jaw a punch right there and break all his pale yellow teeth.

'I'm kidding re!' He laughed as he patted on my back, 'You may go now.'

I didn't waste a second after that. I slung my bag, and this time, I just switched off the monitor. I smiled, thinking about all my unwanted ethics as I walked towards the exit. I still had time to reach the station.

'Deshmukh! You forgot to shut down your PC, I guess.' I heard Muthu calling again. *Bastard! Let me go.*

∞

My phone kept vibrating in my pocket as I jogged my way to the station. Ananya hates to wait. Five minutes is hardly enough to cover a distance of half a mile, considering the fact that most of that distance cuts across the company campus where you won't get any transport, and then you have to cross an eight lane road in the wee hours. As I reached the parking area, I could hear the announcement for our train, though the train was still not in sight. The rest of the distance, I ran at my best speed and only slowed down when I found Ananya at the gate, her eyes flitting from the platform to the road, searching for me.

She put her hands on her hips instead of waving at me. She narrowed her eyes; she wasn't delighted as always on seeing me. She didn't say anything, yet I knew she was angry and wanted an explanation. She would probably ask me why I didn't inform her beforehand, why I kept her waiting, and most importantly, she would definitely ask me why I had ignored her (calls)! I could never win against her in any argument. It was better to try and get away with a sheepish smile! But no, this time, she didn't budge.

'See, I will explain it later. We've got a train to catch!'

'You mean that train,' she pointed at the platform as the train scooted in, 'we just missed it.' She sighed loudly. Well, that was certain indication that I was in big trouble. Gosh! I had let her miss her train.

I turned my face towards her, close enough so I could look into her eyes. 'Just hold my hand and you'll be right in that train.' I didn't wait for her consent, I clutched her wrist in my hand firmly and pulled her along; twenty-five seconds were just about enough.

With her bag swaying wide from her shoulder and those high heels, she struggled, yet she gave it enough to keep pace with me. Moreover, I was not going to leave her hand, so she had no choice but to run with me. Once we reached the door of the compartment, I felt some relief. I grabbed the pole and got in, but a sudden jerk separated us. The train had started moving, I was in it while she was still running on the platform. I moved quickly and hinged my elbow to the pole, leaned out all the way and gave my hand to her.

'Take my hand!' I yelled at her but she was in two minds. I could see the fear in her eyes. The local trains pick up speed quickly, and with every second ticking away, the risk was more. I should have let her stay or simply got off the train myself, but something in me wanted her to come along. Actually, the situation reminded me of that famous scene in the movie *DDLJ*, where like SRK and Kajol, I knew we would make it too. I leaned out further and shouted, 'Trust me, Anu.'

I don't know how it happened. Did I finally catch her hand and yank her in or did she jump in on her own or was there some sort of magic which did it all? Because the only thing I remember is leaning back against the wall of the train with her in my arms. She breathed hard, probably in panic, but I wasn't sure why my heart was sprinting at its best. I held her even more tightly while she lay her head on my chest, her nails hurt as she dug her fingers into my shirt. Suddenly, I realized we were in a train compartment packed with people. I looked around; all those who had shouted at me a moment ago, seeing my stunt, were now looking at us, amused.

'Ananya...Ananya...' I whispered in her ears.

'Am I alive?' she said, still gasping.

'Yes,' I smiled, 'and we're in the train.'

She looked up and glared at me, my hands were still holding her and she was resting heavily against me. She pushed herself away and looked around, suddenly embarrassed. I too felt the same awkwardness, though I thought that the other commuters hardly cared. I mean, couples were such a common sight in Mumbai locals. Then again, were we a couple? No. We had just known each other for some days now. Still, she had already started travelling with me in the general compartment. I would wake up in the morning reading her SMS and would go to bed at night only after sending her a message. And I hated weekends because I couldn't see her. But I still loved Riya and I knew Ananya too had someone in her life. Yeah you guessed it—Sach!

One station later, we got seats. Though we sat next to each other, there was a heavy silence between us. She took the book *Breaking Dawn* out of her bag and started flipping pages; she had forgotten where she had gotten in the story. Of course, with me around she hardly did anything other than talk to me, so it was after a long gap that she was getting back to the world of vampires. I knew she loved the *Twilight* series, she had told me about it the first day itself. And with every passing day, I had only known her more. She had a crush on Yuvraj Singh, she loved Dairy Milk Fruit n Nut, she fasted on Mondays, her mom was twelve years younger than her dad, and *Jaan Tere Naam* was her favourite movie.

Her phone in her rucksack began vibrating but she didn't take it out. I checked the time. It was seven; must be Sach. He called her daily at the same time and she only answered it on his third or fourth attempt. Every day, the same scene repeated. He called, she ignored. Then she picked up, and both of them shouted at each other a bit, and then she disconnected. He would call again but then she would switch off her phone or cut his call. I had asked her many times about it but she always avoided answering. That evening too I was curious, but I didn't dare to ask, I had already done enough damage for the day. I continued playing with my iPad.

'His name is Sachin Masane,' she said, still flipping the pages. 'You didn't ask me today?'

I smiled a tiny smile.

'He is my boyfriend. Rather he was. We broke up few months back,' she continued. I understood why she had always avoided this topic; it must have hurt her a lot. I could see tears welling up in her eyes.

'It's OK. We don't need to talk about that,' I said, and a brief hush followed. She put her phone and book in her bag and sat engrossed in thought. I had actually never seen her this way and I couldn't resist asking her a question, perhaps the most important one.

'Do you love him?'

She shook her head, but the tears that now rolled down her cheeks said a different story. I opted not to probe further.

My station arrived but I didn't want to leave. She sat with her head resting against the window, lost in her memories. She was upset and I couldn't leave her that way. I considered telling her about the new girls who had joined my department in the office, and one of them was really funny. Then I wondered whether I should narrate a page from Subho's diary (I had hacked his system) or simply mimic Muthu. Oh that would surely crack her up! However, she sat lost in her own world. I guessed that she was missing him badly and thought I better not disturb her. I sat quietly beside her, waiting for her to come out of her wonderland.

'Hey!' she exclaimed, 'Nerul?' She had noticed the big signboard at the end of the station as the train moved out.

'I too missed it,' I grinned, anxious to see her reaction to that. She frowned and turned away angrily. Somewhere in my mind, I had expected this of course. I knew she would never read my feelings for her, since after all, I was not supposed to care. I wasn't Sach and she wasn't Riya either.

A couple of minutes later, the train neared Seawoods. I rose from my seat to get down and get back to my apartment. But she held my hand; I turned to her in surprise.

'Boss! Panvel is still a long time away.' She could be so unpredictable, but then, I got what I wanted. A glimpse of her priceless smile.

A Sunny Shady Life

'Don't you think that guy Subho is cute?' Moody said that every time Subho passed by. Moody's real name was Mudrika Kodgire. She was a complete nerd who had spent all her life mugging to score top marks, to get placed in the best company and to impress the best guy around. But I personally felt that she chose the wrong way; she should have groomed her body instead of her brain. Though people said that she was sexy, I had a very different view. God had given her a fair beautiful face; her slim figure complimented her good height. But she sported a terrible hair style and applied coconut oil every alternate day. Her eyebrows were bushy and thick like a rain forest. She smelt like a local Ayurvedic soap and felt proud about it too. She wore the same kind of short kurtas every day, only the colour changed, and I was pretty sure that they all came from her school days. And lastly, she still used Orkut.

'He has a girlfriend,' I glanced at her from the corner of my eye; I could see the sparks in her eyes as they followed Subho till he disappeared into his cubicle.

'How do you know?' Moody questioned me instantly, not out of surprise, but disappointment.

'Well...' I paused trying to think up some reason. Of course I couldn't tell her that I had hacked his system password and read his private files just to kill time in office. Though I didn't do it just to break into his privacy. My system sucked big time with all those administrator permissions. His system was without any such policies; you could access Facebook on his machine or even download Lacie Heart (he had over twenty videos of her saved on his machine).

'What?' She was still waiting.

'I don't know,' I shrugged my shoulders, 'just a wild guess.' I had never shared anything about Subho's files with anyone.

'You may be right, after all, he is a published author,' Richa piped in.

'I honestly don't care whether he is a published author or a porn star,' I said, miffed. I wanted to say this someday to his face, I didn't like him. His flamboyance and his popularity on the floor hurt me. Although younger than me, he had achieved a lot in life.

'You're just jealous!' Richa taunted me with her cruel smile.

Sometimes in life, I fall short of words, but luckily I have a middle finger to convey the message. So, Richa got her reply. I know that was an uncouth response to give to a girl; however, Richa wasn't the kinda girl one would love to have around. She was rude and nasty. God hadn't created her; she was the Devil's own progeny. She had piercings near her eyebrows, flaunted a tattoo on her arm and wore black nailpolish. She had a boy-cut hairdo and went to the gym twice a day. She was tough on emotion and strong on instinct, especially when it came to bashing up people. She habitually greeted and complimented you with cusses, and if you dared to make her angry, then God help you.

'Aaah!' I shrieked in pain as she bent my fingers backward, determined not to leave me until I apologized. Her eyes reflected no mercy and she kept up her killer smile. I knew if I let her have her way a little longer, she would either uproot my finger or simply break it into two. Attack is the best defense, that's what I had learnt in boxing, but instead of a punch, I gave her a pinch on the arm; hard enough for her tattoo to turn red from black instantly, and it was now her turn to scream.

'Oww,' she moaned, and as I drew my hand back and turned around to face my computer, I could see a bunch of geeks gaping at us over their cubicles. I knew I would never be able to explain, so I didn't even try. I unlocked my system and browsed through my emails.

Richa was still standing and I don't know why but she had a big beam on her face, although no one really cared to notice. Amusement is a rare emotion in IT companies and so everyone around was disappointed that it all ended so soon, and that we didn't share the gossip with them. The crowd dispersed and we were back to work. For a moment, I thought nothing had actually happened, but glancing at Richa from the corner of my eyes, I realized something was soon to happen. Something very bad. Richa never forgave!

We didn't even look at each other after that, and Moody wanted us to have lunch together like we did every day. So for her sake, we sat at the same table but on opposite sides. We didn't want to resolve the situation because no one wanted to take the blame. If I had pinched her, she had almost broken my finger. She would naturally say that I showed her the middle finger which was really vulgar, as if I didn't know the level to which she could stoop. And yet, once she started the name calling, I defended myself. She called me 'jealous' and tried to justify it.

'Mean!' I retorted.

'Swine!' she yelled back.

'Bitch!' I screamed.

She held a glass up in the air to hurl it at me while I pulled out the jug, but then I kept it back, thinking she wouldn't mind breaking a chair on my head after that.

'Go to hell,' I turned away.

'Fuck off,' she banged her fist on the table, and the next target of her fist would have been my nose, so I decided to surrender.

'Is everything okay with you guys?' Subho intervened. But both me and Richa didn't give any response, after all the fight had begun thanks to him!

But our Miss Desperate Wannabe offered him a seat which he made a show of accepting. Moody was peering at him as if he were strawberry ice cream with cherry topping. I always wondered what was really so special about this guy. He appeared very weird to me. Over friendly and irritating, poking his nose in everything around him, and if you asked him about one word, he would reply with a whole paragraph, flaunting that he knew everything about everything. His only aim in life was to change his display picture on Facebook daily. Whatever he did he uploaded it there, and then liked and commented on his own updates. He went to a salon twice a year and shaved once a month. His experiments with his looks and dressing were horrible. He came to office in sandals for all seasons and wore a Casio digital watch. And he didn't know that Dark Fantasy was an ice cream and not a condom.

'Sir!' Moody initiated.

'Please don't call me sir. Call me by my name,' he grinned.

'That's really sweet of you,' Moody just couldn't stop blushing. If Richa and I hadn't been there, Moody wouldn't have thought twice to kiss Subho. She was such a *chep*.

'You won the GET of the Year award,' Moody was right on the job.

'Are you telling me or asking me?' he answered sarcastically. *Bloody egoistic jerk!* He went on to narrate his success story in the company and what followed was loud applause and louder giggles from Moody, while Richa and I played with our spoons after lunch, waiting for them to commence their tall tales.

'Even you can win that award if you can work that hard,' Subho said. She seemed super excited at his statements; this is what Moody had wanted to hear all along, that she was simply the best and deserved the best. I just couldn't bear it anymore.

'Yeah! He is so right. You see, it's really not a big deal, you just need to know how to impress our boss, and trust me that's really not difficult for the girls.' I could be mean when required.

'Well if that's what you think, I need to clarify it,' he was a really tough nut to crack. 'I guess to prove your point, you don't need to sleep around with people. The world is very mean and there are just a few good people. And you just have to make the people around you realize that you're among those few,' he had a point blank expression on his face throughout, but his words carried a lot of gravity and felt like a tight slap to me and left me void. I shouldn't have spoken, now I felt ashamed. I couldn't face them and sat on my chair numbed, while they took their plates and left.

∾

They were not talking to me since that scene; they sat in the front row for the training and had not yet logged into their Messenger. I thought they were overreacting, I hadn't actually meant what I said. It was simply a slip of the tongue, that too because I was totally disgusted by Subho's presence. Couldn't they understand this simple fact? But they seemed to not care at all. They murmured and giggled all through the session. In the tea break, Subho joined them, I had come along but they just ignored me. *Even I don't care, go to hell*, I thought to myself.

Why is it that I do nice things for people all the time and they never notice, but one mistake and it's never forgotten, I wondered. *I don't need them, I don't need them,* I repeated these lines over and over in my head every time I thought about them. I tried to concentrate on the training module on my monitor but it didn't help. These were the only friends I had in Mumbai and without them, I felt an emptiness inside me. I did care for them and need them, madly.

As the day's session ended, I thought about talking to them, maybe just a small apology, although even that much was really difficult for me. I had to accept my fault first I realized, and only then it would be easy for me to go ahead. But before I could make up my mind about what to do, they were already gone. I trudged behind them reluctantly and found myself at the place where it had all started. The food court. They went on to sit at a table and I pondered on whether to approach them or not. I was wrong, I accepted it. But I found I couldn't take any steps forward. Did I fear being snubbed or was it that stupid ego in me again? I didn't know. I watched them from a distance, they ordered coffee, and they ordered three. Damn! Three coffees! So it wasn't that bad. They still wanted me! I rejoiced within and ran ahead. I wanted them too. For my own sake. For my smiles. For my happiness.

'Richa! Moody!' I was panting when I reached them. They glared at me in silence. 'I'm sorry for the afternoon,' I said and sat down on the lone empty chair.

'Really?' Moody asked. I nodded convincingly as I pulled my coffee closer and took a sip.

'It's OK!' Moody smiled. I too beamed. I looked at Richa, she still wouldn't budge.

'Oh! C'mon now. See, he is apologizing,' Moody insisted and Richa finally managed a tiny smile.

'OK! But better mind it next time,' it wasn't a warning, it was a threat and I had no choice but to smile.

'Jo hukum mere akka,' I toasted my coffee.

'Very funny!' Richa retorted, 'By the way, this coffee was for Subho and not for you. He is coming.'

For a moment, we all looked at each other and burst out laughing. Everything between us was alright again.

ა

'Let's party!' Richa announced and everyone followed her in chorus. Subho and Pritam, who was more popularly called Dummy, had also joined us. There was this private joke that floated around in our department whenever we began meetings, *to put our phones on Pritam mode.*

He had joined the company with Subho (I always wondered how he had cracked the interview), he was a core Mechanical guy but he didn't say anything at the interview and ended up being a system administrator. He worked day and night but didn't speak much and never got good ratings. He was the most knowledgeable person in the department but didn't ever speak up for himself and Subho won the best GET award. He loved Moody right from the first day but again didn't say anything and...

Well, let's keep that in suspense for now.

OK! Back to everyone. Their excitement and enthusiasm scared me. I checked my watch, it was 5.45. I wished whatever their plans were, they didn't meant to implement them right away. Ananya had already called me twice in the training room. I had cut her calls and she had messaged saying that she had great news to share. She would be expecting me after six and no way was I going to let her down.

'Should we go to the executive lounge or some restaurant outside the campus?' Subho was such a pain in neck.

'Why don't we think about this tonight and decide tomorrow?' I suggested and everyone gave me a cold stare.

'Moody, won't you be late getting home? Your dad will kill you if he comes to know that you were partying with us!' I tried the other way out.

'Well…' she thought for a while. 'I'll lie at home that I had extra work in office,' she was smiling again, looking at Subho. *Bloody despo!*

'What's your problem?' Richa asked me.

'I'm just very tired,' I replied.

'Is it?' she said, teasing me. She had sensed the truth. 'I guess you're not too tired for your chick.'

'Richa!' I yelled at her. 'Mind it!'

'Mind what? Will you explain?'

'Why the hell do you need to drag Ananya into everything?'

'Oh! Her name is Ananya,' Subho cut in. 'I saw both of you many times together in the train. Is she your girlfriend?'

'No. She isn't. She is just a friend,' I explained.

'Then why are you so concerned? Is she so important to you that you're ditching all your friends just to give her company? Don't you value us? It's just one evening we're asking for,' Moody was such a drama queen. Though she had asked me a question, I was just supposed to blindly nod in agreement.

'Yes! I'm coming. Let's party,' I uttered, unable to bear the *emotional atyachar* further.

So we went to a restaurant outside our campus. We seated ourselves and ordered ice cream and cold coffee. This was what they meant by a party? I mean, if not black currant, we would have got kulfi, if not cappuccino, we would have got Coke in our food court itself, then why this bloody outing! I felt frustrated sitting with them there. I checked my watch. Five minutes to six. I pictured her packing her stuff, and sure enough, my phone beeped with a message: *Let's go*. As my phone beeped, everybody stopped whatever they were doing and glared at me as if they had all been waiting for this moment; they wanted to see my reaction. I picked up my phone and rose from my chair.

'I need to make a call,' I said.

'So, you're waiting for our permission,' Richa smirked and everyone lauded her with a roar of laughter. Of course, the first thing that came to my mind was to show her my middle finger but the morning saga was still fresh in my mind. I excused myself from the comedy circus to call Ananya.

'Hey! Where are you?' She picked up even before I could hear it ring at the other end; she had been waiting for me.

'I'm out with friends. Can't come today, you go ahead,' I said.

'What?!' she took a long breath. 'Pathetic!' she said. 'How could you do that? I'm waiting for you here. I had told you that I had this great news to share with you but you still went out with your friends,' she paused. 'That's fine, I don't care. Now, I have to walk all the way alone because I let my friends go ahead, because I wanted to tell you first. Damn! You and your friendship, pathetic!' She cut the call.

∽

I was waiting for my train after the so-called party. The station looked a bit different; I couldn't believe this was the very place where I boarded my train twice a day, where I spent such a lot of time either waiting for my train or with Ananya. The bench where we sat daily looked unfamiliar. I had actually never noticed that it was grayish-green in colour, its legs were rusted and crooked. There was a pigeon's nest on the wall just behind the bench and I noticed it for the first time. I kept glancing towards the gate every now and then, only to realize that she wouldn't come, she was gone already. It was 7.15, she must have reached home. Well no, she must only have reached the HDFC circle; she always talked with me on her way home. I wanted to call her but knowing she might still be angry, dropped her a message instead—*Message me when you reach home.*

I checked my cell phone every few minutes after that, but there was no reply from her. I had got a window seat but was really not interested in the view outside; anyway there wasn't anything fascinating to see other than the packed evening crowd on station platforms or the never ending slums. Even my iPad failed to entertain me, NFS and Jay Sean just could not keep me from thinking about her. Whether it was Richa's taunts, Moody's caring or Ananya's company, I was so accustomed to all of them that just the thought of letting go of any of them seemed apocalyptic. It was like they all had come into my life as a package and any missing link would spoil everything else in my new world. I needed them all; just to keep myself alive during my time in Mumbai.

I dialled her number as soon as I got off the train. At the most, she would shout at me again or would not take my call, I thought. What was there to be afraid of? After all, she was a normal girl and was just a friend, not my girlfriend, I told myself.

'Hello!' she answered my call.

'Hi Ananya,' I said, 'have you reached home?'

'Yep! Why are you asking?'

'Well! Am I not supposed to?'

'Nothing like that but why suddenly?'

'I was worried. I mean I let you go alone today.'

'So what? Dear, I've been travelling alone since the age of eleven and anyway, you won't be there for me always.' *When it came to bullying, nobody could beat her.*

'I'm sorry. I won't do it again, I promise,' I pleaded.

'What's wrong with you Gautam? Are you all right?' Finally she showed some concern.

'Yeah! I am. I missed you a lot.'

'I too missed you, dear.'

'Anyway, tell me what was the good news? You wanted to tell me something?'

She told me that her request to change her work profile had been accepted. She explained everything about it but all that stuff about accounts went over my head, I just wanted to hear her sweet voice till eternity. And we continued talking, I don't know how long. We disconnected only when her Mom yelled out to her to put the phone down and have dinner. I too went into the kitchen. Kantabai had made some mixed vegetable curry which I didn't dare taste. I felt full just looking at it. I pulled out a beer from the fridge and went to the balcony. Kingfisher and Goldflake make quite a combination to give a lone soul company; I took a puff and a sip alternately, sitting on the chair, staring at the night sky. That was my favourite pastime those days. A few minutes later, Ananya messaged me goodnight and I replied, but I wasn't really going to bed. I opened Facebook.

I would stalk Riya's profile every night. Unlike Orkut, Facebook doesn't tell you who visited your profile. I had always been tempted to send her a Friend Request or just a message saying hello, but I knew the moment she saw my name, she would block me. The distance between us had grown so wide that even the sky above us looked different to us now.

Of late, I noticed a trend in her display pictures. She posted those random pictures available on the internet, relating to love in general, and even if she uploaded pictures of herself, they had to be ones where she was always blushing. It was her way of telling the world that she was seeing someone. She had done the same when she was with me. That 'Single' status was finally gone from her profile.

Six months was all it had taken for her to get over a seven year long relationship and move on to another guy in her life.

Nothing lasts forever, I realized. Especially love.

∽

Corporate Atyachar

From being a carefree rich brat to a corporate slave, I made the transition in just thirty days. Why not, after all, I had been working really hard on those nine commandments that every engineer promises to follow before joining any IT company:

I have already enjoyed my life in childhood.

I love tension.

I don't want to spend time with my friends (I hate them).

I love night duty.

I love to work on Sundays and holidays.

I want to take revenge on myself.

I don't want to get married before 30 years of age.

I want to study until my death.

I don't want hair on my head.

Simply put, the life of an IT professional really sucks. And it wasn't just me who was unhappy or frustrated; peeping over my cubicle, I could see many useless (useful for clients) heads of other labourers, toiling away day and night for their daily pizzas and burgers. Here in IT, most people think, 'Is this really what I want to do in life?', but the very next minute they get a ping from their manager or TL regarding the task update, and then they try to recollect, 'Where am I'. This is a common story for all those who work in IT, and yet, we comfort ourselves in the thought that we are 'surviving', rather 'growing'. But how? This question, of course, possesses the same gravity as that of a question on the Indian economy: How does the economy grow? Exactly!

Early to bed, early to rise makes a man healthy, wealthy and wise;

I knew why I was none of them. The day started with an 8.30 alarm ring because my tummy needed that much time to slowly digest the tandoori chicken and beer of the previous night. So after my beauty sleep, I got up and went straight to office. Yes guys! You caught me. I deliberately avoided saying that I had a bath and all, because those were optional activities and depended on the circumstances. You see, deodorant companies had made life so simple.

Once in office, I spent lots of time on Gtalk, Facebook (through proxy sites) and tea breaks, apart from attending meetings and trainings. And yes! I did some work too, if I still had time. Well, about my work, being a software tester, my job was to run a few tools on some applications and look for bugs or glitches in them. Yeah! It does sound simple and trust me, it really was that easy, although it could lull a person to sleep with its hypnotically ugly monotony; luckily, we had a large coffee maker which poured out hot chocolate too, though I wish it poured out beer. Everything in the office was so dull and the routine made me sometimes feel as if I was in a jail, where weekends meant bail. Life became a long wait from one Saturday to another, because after Monday and Tuesday, even my calendar said WTF.

The other thing I observed was that in the IT world, you always need to be able to elaborate on simple things in a complicated manner; if you can do that, you have a really good future. Here, you will find people working day and night without looking at Saturdays and Sundays on the calendar, and also people who come to office at 11.30 a.m. and are right there, outside the premises, waiting for the bus at 6 p.m. sharp. This is one weird industry, where two people in the same position with the same experience can differ drastically in salaries. It's all about Darwin's theory—survival of the fittest and being fittest here means being the mean, selfish, greedy and politico type. Sometimes, I too asked myself the question, 'How the hell did I end up here?'

But you know, it is a fun industry, to be part of long calls and important meetings, to relish the never-affordable food in client parties, to play pool and TT in every two-hour break after working for an hour, to enjoy the weekend sleeping in for three days (yes, I have included Friday too!), to work hard outside the office in your 'bench' period, banging your head over the forever-changing requirements and never-ending client expectations. And at the end of the long wait of thirty days, finally the most awaited SMS, from the bank—*Your salary has been credited to your account*—that made everything worth it. Life is really good here.

∞

I hated those progress review meetings. They were not only boring and dull but also unduly prolonged, continuing beyond work hours. Moreover, they always brought bad news like errors in submitted modules, criticism from clients and increased targets. The projects were always big and went on for months or even more than a year sometimes, and the IT sector being a fast-changing environment, it would become difficult to stay connected with our objectives and agendas through the duration of the project. Application changes, technology changes, requirement changes, and more often, people change—all in a matter of days. But what was more disgusting was the fact that being freshers, we were expected to be attentive throughout the torment, take notes and not open our mouths even for talking or yawning. Sick!

'I'm under pressure from the management, why are we not able to close this project yet?' Our HOD, Mr Bose demanded, aghast at seeing the progress report. Our conference room was in panic mode, there were graphs projected on the wall, heaps of paper on the table, and laptops processing away, but they all said the same thing essentially—*you're so fucked up*.

'We are almost done with it, just waiting for the transaction module to be completed,' Muthu defended.

'Waiting for whom?' Mr Bose questioned.

'Vendors!' Muthu answered. There was stunned silence after that. He had hit a bingo; the madness in Mr Bose's mind seemed to have hit a road block. The tensed faces around got some brief respite while we three, however, were still clueless about the whole hungama.

'What do they want now?'

'More money.'

'You know that's not possible. We can't do that till year end.'

'Well, I'm sorry to say then, we will have to wait,' that wasn't an answer that Mr Bose would've liked to hear, and that too, coming from Muthu. However, Muthu was absolutely right, their hands were tied by company policy and nothing else could have been done. They had to wait.

The meeting was dispersed. Everybody went to their respective workstations. Mr Bose was still sitting in the conference room, looking deflated. Being an ex-army man, it was hard for him to digest defeat. Perhaps, he was fully aware of the consequences. The company was in bad shape and under-performance could bring on a lot of trouble. It was a time of recession. Employee pay cuts were so common in the IT sector; though Mr Bose was safe, the sword had to fall on someone's head, and that's what was bothering him because he loved his team like his own family. On the other hand, Muthu seemed pleased; if all the odds were stacked against Mr Bose, he still had a chance to retain his cabin and rule, which was what he always wanted. But being more experienced, Mr Bose was preferred ahead of Muthu, for his extra calibre and charismatic personality. Of course, Mr Bose was a great man, and probably, the most handsome boss on earth (Moody told me this on the first day, that she had been disappointed when she discovered he was happily married with two children). It always hurt Muthu to see how popular Mr Bose was, so when the whole lot of people seemed worried about the possibilities, Muthu just made his way to the coffee maker, smiling. If there were categories in assholes, Muthu was a category in himself.

I logged into my system and opened the files I had saved concerning this project. Though it seemed mere stupidity for me to even try anything, I mean, I was just a fresher and if all the big minds had given up, what difference could I make? But still, I wanted to give it an honest try, not that I respected Mr Bose very much and couldn't see him like that, sad and tensed, but because I hated Muthu very very much and couldn't see him like that, happy and smiling. May he fall while walking and break a few front teeth, I muttered. At least I wouldn't have to bear the ugly sight of him smiling nonstop then.

'Subho!' I reluctantly went up to him; he was the only person who could help.

'What?' he responded, busy fiddling with his mobile phone.

'I need to talk to you.'

'Just wait a minute, I'm sending an important mail,' he said.

'See, I want to talk about this portal.'

'What about it?'

'If it's really that important, why don't we do it ourselves?' I said. He gave me this blank look. 'I mean, we do have developers.'

'That's not our job. It was outsourced to vendors.'

'Does it matter? We can do that ourselves here and save a lot of money for the company. It will even help us learn, don't you think?' I reasoned.

'Dude! I do understand but see, we are already loaded with work. We don't have time for extra work. Why don't you ask Ali? He would be happy to help you,' he added with a smirk. As if I didn't know how much work he had. I knew that he wasn't really sending any mail; he was uploading a photo of himself, taken in the conference room, on Facebook. *Jerk!*

☙

Let me tell you a story now.

Once a young lady was walking down a street. She stopped at a small house where an old man was sitting on a rocking chair on the porch. She was so amazed to see this man merrily rocking away on his chair and smoking a cigarette that she couldn't resist talking to him.

'Hello sir!' she greeted and the man gestured to her with a broad smile. 'It's really such a pleasure to see you, so happy and enjoying the evening. At your age, when people become so cynical about life, you look so cheerful and radiant. May I please know the secret of your happiness?'

The man smiled and said, 'Well pretty lady, I have been following a strict routine for quite some time now. I start my day with a bottle of beer to kill the hangover of last night. I drink six pegs of vodka neat, by noon, and go to bed only after finishing half a whiskey bottle. I smoke two packets of cigarettes daily and chew tobacco when I run out of money. I also do drugs occasionally. I sleep never before 4 a.m. I love junk food and I never exercise.'

'What's your age?' the lady interrupted him, shocked by now.

'Twenty-six,' he said smiling.

The lady fainted.

And that man was our Ali. He was the phantom of our department. four years in the company and nobody knew anything about him other than his name. His family, his education, his native place, all remained a mystery. His quietness made people suspicious. He never socialized with anyone; he talked only about work, didn't use a cell phone and didn't have a Facebook account. No coffee, no tea, no breakfast, no lunch; he took breaks from work only to smoke and pee. He played *Metallica* in full volume on head-phones to avoid being disturbed by anyone. And if anyone happened to share a word with him, it had to be about either Java or sex. Some called him a jerk, some said he was gay, some rumoured that he was a terrorist, and Subho believed he was an alien who survived on photosynthesis, and trust me, it was possible since nobody had seen him eating anything ever. Man, was he a vampire...I wondered.

'Hey Ali!' I called. He ignored me completely, he was typing some codes.

'Hey!' I shook him and he reacted as if he had felt an electric shock. He glanced at me but his fingers were still moving over his keyboard.

'Yes!' he beamed.

'I need your help for my module,' I said.

'Ya sure, but you see I'm busy right now. Let's discuss it in detail after office hours.' And with that, his grin spread by a few centimetres and his brief affectionate gaze gave me the scare of a lifetime. *Hell with the portal! I don't mind Muthu ruling the whole company; I would never dare to come to Ali again.*

∽

When I finally shut down my laptop, it was four in the morning. But did I care for the time? The work wasn't finished and yet I had to stop; it wasn't me who was tired, my laptop finally gave up. It had been up and running for a straight 60 hours. I typed codes all night and put them to test while leaving for office in the morning. And when I returned, I was welcomed by success sometimes, but debug or runtime errors most of the time. However, those failures only told me about the mistakes I needed to avoid, and with every passing hour that I spent before my laptop, I only bettered my skills. Though I can't say that it was only me who was concerned about this portal working out, Ali turned out to be a genuine help and more importantly, a thorough genius. After office, we would spend hours discussing (Richa always covered for me while Ali was around) the details of our progress and what to implement next. And one evening, when I returned home, I saw my laptop flashing a request for my employ ID and password. *Everest conquered!* My endless labour, sleepless nights and gallons of coffee to keep my eyes open had finally borne fruit. The portal was ready.

Although it did seem stupid to even tell Muthu about the portal, I actually demonstrated it to him. He appeared more shocked than pleased at my efforts. I still remember the day of my interview. He had called me dumb and was not in favour of selecting me, when I gave a blank look on being asked what was the Biot-Savart's law, (I still don't know what it is!). So in a way, I did have an idea of what to expect from him.

'You made this?' he oppugned. See, I was absolutely right. *Asshole! If not me then who?* I smiled at him benignly.

'It actually seems good,' he mused, 'but there're a few big glitches.'

'Really?' I snapped.

'Yes! I don't think this is user friendly. See, there are very few shortcut links and also this one doesn't save the passwords.'

'Why do you want it to save passwords?' I argued. 'I made it that way purposely, to secure privacy, and I also feel if not user friendly, it's at least engineer friendly. There won't be any problem.'

'Whatever!' he retorted. 'I still need to test it thoroughly before approving it.'

'Fine!' I grumbled.

'By the way, Deshmukh! Is green a colour for such an important thing?'

'Does it make any difference?' I snorted. 'Would you have been happy if I had painted the portal pink?'

He just returned a broad smile, the kind of smile I hated more than anything else in this world. There was no use arguing, it would never be approved. This office politics is everywhere. Seniors never let their juniors go ahead. Subho was right, it was not my job and I shouldn't have worked on it. Still, seeing my efforts going in vain made me feel let down, and I quietly retreated to my desk and continued to work on testing crap applications. I was numb the rest of the time, hardly ate anything for lunch, and didn't even talk to anyone. Richa wasn't arguing, Moody wasn't smiling, Subho wasn't giving gyan and Pritam wasn't doing anything (anyway he did nothing all the time); my friends had always understood me well and their silence only meant they supported me. They knew I was down in the dumps and no words could heal my pain for the time being.

When I came back to the floor after lunch, there was some celebration going on. Everyone had gathered at the centre table, a cake was brought in, people were congratulating each other, and Mr Bose was ready for yet another yawning speech. I looked at Subho but he too was oblivious to the proceedings.

'Good afternoon everyone! We've done it!' Mr Bose announced excitedly and everyone responded with a loud roar of cheers. Something really big had happened!

'We've shown the management of what we are capable of,' he

continued with his prowess over words. I felt as if aliens had attacked us and Mr Bose was there to motivate us to fight for our land, women and children. I tell you this man really would have made a brilliant politician. But the problem with him was that he easily got carried away, twenty minutes up and most of the people still did not know what the speech was all about. He finally came to the point when the crowd started showing signs of apathy.

'The portal is ready. The project is closed.' This statement by him almost made me skip a heartbeat. I couldn't believe my ears; I looked at my friends, they were smiling at me. Whoa! It was finally approved.

'Muthu and his team, great work!' he joyfully exclaimed. This time, I almost got a mini heart attack. That name MUTHU hit my ears like a bomb exploding and echoed in my mind, while a round of applause and claps followed. Muthu almost danced his way to shake hands with Mr Bose and that fucking smile was still plastered all over his face. Man, office politics could get so dirty! Pritam held me back from bursting out in protest, his hand pressing down on my shoulder.

Muthu limited his tale to very, very few words when he was asked how it happened. I had to admire his courage that even after doing nothing, he managed to take all the accolades, looking straight into my eyes.

'Well, you see the portal is very simple in appearance and quite complex in application, so as to limit its use to engineers. It doesn't save any password to avoid misuse. And most importantly, it's green in colour, to show our support to the environment,' he grinned.

He went on with his demonstration, feeding in the username and the default password but the LED screen flashed a login error. He tried again but my baby still didn't give him access. His repeated unsuccessful attempts made people mock at him, a few even taunted him aloud and Muthu gave them a dirty look in return. But nobody feared him, even Mr Bose's presence couldn't save him from embarrassment. He looked at me, and though he didn't say anything, I knew he wanted help. *Why should I help,* was my first thought, but I also couldn't see my baby fail in its first steps. So I walked up to the system and typed the password.

Access granted.

Welcome user.

Before I turned around, I could already hear big cheers and loud whistles, all meant for me. I gazed at Muthu confidently with my eyes reflecting my triumph and his remorse. He had done everything right to credit my labours to his name and had almost gotten away with it, but he had forgotten to turn Caps Lock off while typing the password. Hard luck! Fortune favours only the brave.

Those Were the Days

One hour was simply not enough for me to return, I was very well aware of that and yet I took the risk. Was it right or wrong, I didn't want to decide then. I couldn't make the choice; I was going out with Ananya and then coming back for my friends. I guess only Superman could make it in time. I knew I had to say a *no* to Ananya, but then I had already done that once for them. One more time would not have been a big deal. But I had one hour in hand. I would manage it, I assured myself.

'Armaan!' she murmured, peering at a little boy who was sitting opposite us in the train.

'What?' I inquired.

She took a deep breath, a long story was to follow, and I dared not yawn at all, no matter how *pathetic* it would be.

'I am just fascinated by this name. I will name my boy the same,' she was still smiling, looking at the little boy.

Hats off to this creation of God. Girls. When we boys don't even know what we will do for the evening, girls think all the way to what they will name their kids. What should I say? Pathetic, maybe! I could only smile at her weakly.

'Hey! I got something for you,' she put her hand inside her bag, searching for something. She couldn't find it. 'It must be there somewhere.' She started taking out all her stuff to find it. Sunglasses, lipstick, comb, hair clip, water bottle, face powder, a little mirror, eye liner, napkin, charger, toothbrush…

'Toothbrush?' I was astounded.

'Hah! In case of emergency.'

'Emergency?'

'What if I had to stay back at some friend's place, so just in case.' I shook my head.

'There it is!' she found it. A little card, a friendship card.

'Life is a big party with friends like you around,' I read out.

'Isn't it cute?'

I nodded. I was grinning ear to ear. 'Hey! You didn't write your name anywhere.'

'Oh shit! I forgot.'

'Don't you have a pen in your bag?'

She shook her head. 'Well, give it to me,' she snatched the card, looked at it once, then took out her lipstick, applied it and kissed the card on one side.'

'I guess this one is even better,' I took the card back and kept it carefully in my bag.

She was blushing. 'It's hot here, let's stand at the door.'

It may sound weird to those who have travelled by Mumbai locals, to give up seats just like that, but trust me, the feeling is extremely refreshing, when after a hectic day in the office, you have a girl to hang out with you, you feel simply blessed. I was standing on the footboard holding the bar on the wall and hanging half out, while she stood between me and the door. The train shot to speed in seconds once it started. The inertia pushed us backwards and I rested myself on the pole in the middle, she was leaning against my chest and her long hair was fluttering into my face (she had switched to Garnier from Head & Shoulders, I noticed). The wind was so harsh that it almost tore at the buttons and blew my shirt away but I still didn't want to move an inch and it wasn't only because of the *Ananya effect*. Whether it was the fast passing stations, the narrow tunnels or the long and dodgy bridges, one little careless move or even a slip and you're straight in hell, but who really cared? I was already in heaven; I had no fear in me and I howled like a wolf all through the ride, trying to match the sound of the wind. She was calm and smiling silently; I was concerned for her safety. I pulled my hand from the roof and held the door to guard her; my hands touched hers and I quickly slipped my hand further above. She covered my hand with her palm and held on tight. The warmth in her touch made my heart beat faster; I wondered whether she knew what she was doing. She was still leaning on me, smiling. The train was just about to reach the last stop and so there were very few commuters. The train was passing through a dark woody stretch. Maybe all those things gave me some blind confidence or courage, I don't know, but I drew my face close enough to rest my chin on her shoulder. I could feel her breath and she was breathing hard too. What next, I thought. The train was rounding a curve; she struggled to keep her balance. I reacted immediately; I put my other arm around her waist and pulled her closer. She was secure in my arms. The comfortable silence between us said a lot, but *where were we heading? What did she want? Was everything alright between us?* Such questions came fast and furious, with no answers to follow though. Everything seemed confusing and I wanted to know how to end the turmoil in my head. And finally, at the long whistle of the train, the moment was over. I looked outside; I could see the lights on the station platforms. We moved away from the door for the commuters who had gathered to get down but when we stepped out, we were holding hands.

At the end of the platform I stood, watching her go. I waited till she crossed the bridge, she didn't look back. I walked out of the station with the train scene replaying in my mind. I had been to heaven and back. I took my cell phone out to check the time. I saw two missed calls, Subho had called me, but when you're going at that speed, you have no friends. I had just twenty minutes to go. I ran towards the taxi stand, my train back was still ten minutes away. But considering it was peak hour, was a cab the right choice, I wondered. Ten minutes was a lot of time to waste, I figured.

'Khoperkhairne?' I asked the cab driver.

'Three hundred,' he said.

'I will give you five hundred but I'll drive,' and I showed him my driving license.

He gave me a blank look.

'OK! Here it is,' I almost threw the note at his face. 'Now move.'

I opened the driver's door and eased myself in. The driver still looked bewildered as he slipped to the side seat but the extra bucks had shut his mouth.

'Put on your seat belt,' I commanded as I stepped on the accelerator.

∾

I pulled the hand brake at top speed; the locked tires skidded hard on the ground making a loud squealing sound and spun the car at 180 degrees. Passers by stopped to have a look, then saw it was neither an accident nor a stunt; I was just in a hurry. When I looked sideways at the driver, he had a new hairstyle. The expression on his face reflected the horror he had just experienced, leaving him dumb and numb. I can bet my kidneys on it that he would never give his taxi ever again to anybody, not even for a million rupees! I stepped out of the car in style; my phone told me that I still had three minutes, enough for me to walk from the company main gate to my department.

It was actually Subho's big day; he was to be honoured at an event held in his school and each one of us had contributed in some way to prepare him for the grand moment ahead. We were all invited for the function and couldn't wait to join Subho. Moody was going to miss out on all the action because of her strict dad. Richa told me that Moody had cried in the washroom; after all, we all knew what Subho meant to her. All the more reason I was determined to make it a very special and memorable day for him. And had a big surprise waiting for him in the parking lot.

'Guys! Here it is,' I pointed at my car, 'we are going in this.'

They couldn't take their eyes off my Volkswagen beauty, their jaws almost dropped to the ground seeing this one car that stood out among all the cars in the parking lot.

'Dude! That's a Beetle,' Ali exclaimed in astonishment.

'I'm not paying for it,' Subho paused to take a deep breath. 'I mean I couldn't pay for it anyhow. Where did you hire it from?'

'Don't worry, you don't have to pay anything. It's my car,' I smiled.

For a moment, they all gave me a blank look and then went back to gawking at my *Rampyari* in awed fascination.

'Ha! If this car belongs to you, then I must be Batman,' Subho laughed it off.

'I'm serious bro, that's my car,' I defended without a smile this time, but they still didn't look convinced.

'I guess the drive will be long enough for me to explain my story,' I said sheepishly.

Driving to Subho's hometown, I thought the journey would never end! *No way can you call yourself a Mumbaikar, Subho, your place is way beyond the outskirts of the city*, I mused as I drove. I wondered how he managed to travel all that distance every day and still be cheerful at work. The ride was long enough for me to tell them my entire story. Hell, I could have told them stories about ten generations of my family! When we finally reached the destination, I knew that had I driven a few more kilometres, I would have been able to say hello to my mom in Pune.

'Gosh! You mean you are *the* Gautam Deshmukh?!' Richa exclaimed every few minutes. And I would nod and smile.

'I've read about you and your family in magazines and papers. Wow! I know Gautam Deshmukh,' she went on excitedly.

'Yeah! We thought you were just a geek and you happen to be a prince who is here to prove himself and win back his princess. It's all like a fantasy,' Subho said sarcastically.

'It's not just me; everyone has their own story to tell, don't they Subho?' I teased.

'What do you mean?' He raised his eyebrow.

'I know that there is someone in your life and I hope it's not Moody.'

'C'mon, you must be crazy to think like that,' he protested immediately. Of course, from his diary I knew that it wasn't Moody. I only wanted to use her name so that he would spill the mystery of his diary girl.

'She was with me in high school. I love her since then.'

'Does she even know about your feelings?'

'Yeah! She does, but the problem is that she doesn't feel the same way for me.' He paused, as if struck by a stream of old memories. 'She is in Tampa, somewhere in the US,' he added. Looking at him only reaffirmed my own thoughts. Love has the power to both create and destroy people.

His mood went cold after that and he sat looking outside the window impassively. I truly understood what he was going through; I had read about it all in his diary—his passion, his emotions, his pain, his songs. And his endless wait, eight years was a really long time. That girl must be really dumb to not value such enduring love.

I looked in the rear mirror. Mr Dumbo (Pritam) and Mr Enigma (Ali) were fast asleep on either side of Richa, their heads resting on her shoulders. She had this expression of disgust written all over her face, looking so different from her usual bubbly self.

'So what's your story, girl?' I asked her. She smiled although her expression was serious. But I was pretty sure whatever she would narrate, no matter how severe, could only bring a smile to our dull faces.

'I hate being myself,' she said in a heavy voice. Subho and I were surprised at her words, but instead of interrupting her or making a joke out of it, we remained silent and listened to her attentively.

'Like every other girl on this planet, I too love to dress up, put on make-up, try out fancy hairstyles and woo guys. But no matter how hard I try, I will remain an ugly hag. It really hurts when no one gives me a second glance. If I was born dark, is it my fault? Why can't people go beyond looks? So I decided long ago that I am better off opting out of this race. Why should I even care for what others think? Over the years, this attitude has really worked for me; I have learnt many ways to keep myself happy. But now my parents want me to get married and you see, I have already paraded for boys' families four times. But each guy has rejected me for my dark complexion. It's kinda like racism, you know? I feel so insulted that now, I just don't want to get married. I'm happy like this only.' She almost sobbed as she spoke that last sentence.

This thing called love had touched everyone's life in some way or the other, I realized. Love is cruel, it only makes everything complicated and turns life into hell. And still we all want to fall in love. Why? Because love is an experience that makes us feel completely alive, completely new, where every sense is heightened, every emotion is magnified, our everyday reality is immaterial and we constantly feel as if we are flying in heaven. It may not last a lifetime, or a year, or even a day, but that doesn't diminish its value because we are left with memories, both good and bad, that we treasure for the rest of our lives. Oh, to be in love!

The rest of the evening was simply great. Subho gave an awesome speech with no relevance to reality. I mean, he was such a lazy guy that he had never woken up early in the morning even during exams. He had always passed papers by stealing notes from toppers, and when it came to his track record for behaviour, he had once written in his book that two of his teachers were lesbians and twice, he had been suspended for low attendance. So you can imagine his reputation. Yet, there we were, clapping for him and those little kids from his school who looked up to him as their mentor!

∽

Dear Riya,

You may have noticed that for a few days now, I've been writing a lot about my new friends here. That's because they are simply the coolest people on earth. Each and every moment spent with them is worth cherishing all my life and I feel I'm blessed to have them around, just the way you made me feel when you were with me. I miss you so much baby!

We are all very different in many aspects; we would never even have looked at each other if we hadn't met that way. But then that's the beauty of friendship, we would miss out on knowing such lovely people in life if we didn't dare to talk to strangers. It is these differences in people that create magic in our lives, just like light is meaningful only in relation to darkness and truth presupposes error. I know these are heavy words to digest, and why not, especially when you're in the company of an author (Subho), a perfectionist (Moody), a lady Rambo (Richa) and a genius (Ali). Together, we make the Super Six. I guess I missed someone. Add Pritam to the list, he exists too. Ha ha ha.

Bye for now. Gonna be waiting for your reply as always and please don't disappoint me as always.

I love you.

∽

I typed my password and hit Enter. As my computer loaded the personal settings, I glanced at others out of the corner of my eyes; Richa was the closest. Her system was asking for her password but I realized that I was the first to cross the finish line.

'I won!' I declared. We were playing *Whose PC boots first.*

We had discovered quite a number of games in the office, like *Whose PC can run maximum number of applications at a time* and *Who can aim maximum number of coffee cups into the dustbin*. Subho once said that he could write a book on *1001 innovative ways to waste time in office*. But seriously, office gossip is where the real fun of work life lies. No matter what the opening topic, it always ends on promotions and increments, things that never happen when one sticks to the same company for years. Perhaps, most of the time, people are busy investigating who's next to leave or join.

'Attention everyone!' Mr Bose called out. Sensing a big announcement ahead, we all rose from our seats and gathered at the centre of the room.

'I need to introduce you to our new colleague, Mr Samir Hariharan from Banglore.' And then Mr Bose narrated a dozen stories of *Mr Hariharan's* life, starting from his childhood hero (Shaktiman) to his latest crush (Kajjal Agrawal) while the poor chap just stood there, smiling sheepishly. He seemed classy in appearance. He was probably one of those guys who only wore ironed underwear and socks, and when he spoke, it seemed as if he had already rehearsed his lines many times. Six feet tall, dark and handsome, he probably wore only top brands. The costly Rolex on his wrist indicated how much he must have cost to the company.

'He is a gold medalist and topper from his class. He has handled many big projects and has been awarded for his work. When I heard about him, I knew he is the best guy to handle our network coverage project.'

And my mind promptly went, *Gosh! No. I hate you Mr Bose for saying this*. We all looked at each other at the same instant with expressions of despair and turned to look at Moody. She was already smiling, gawking at her latest muse. The touch of mirth in her eyes seemed to say that she had been waiting for this very guy all her life. Basically, the same feeling that once resonated in her heart for Subho and God knows how many more before him. No matter we called her Moody.

Welcome to Moody's world, Mr Samir Hariharan.

Of Course I Love You

The day after Diwali night...

Was 2.00 a.m. that late for a software engineer? Maybe I was just tired after the hectic day...Or was something bothering me? I wasn't sure. I felt strange stalking Riya's Facebook profile that night and realized that my heart was not in it one hundred percent. I wanted to write to her, but knew that it would make no difference to her. She didn't care anymore, even if it was breaking me within. Anyway, what would I have written? That I chased a girl, fought with her friends, later danced with her in the rain and then dropped her home. That she had asked me whether I loved her and I had almost said yes.

I slept fitfully for a while; if not my mind, at least my body was tired. My mind kept replaying vision after vision of Ananya. I was pleased seeing her in my dreams like this, but suddenly reality hit and I woke up in the middle of night in a sweat. *What was she doing to me?* I asked myself aloud and looked for an answer in my phone. But her phone had remained switched off from the time she had vanished from the station.

She did send me a message in the morning, wishing me a happy Diwali, but that was a forwarded message meant for everyone. I knew that I wouldn't meet her for a while since the next two days were a holiday. Waiting so long was a dreadful option, so I wondered whether I should just go visit her at her house. Of course, I barely knew her address. All I knew was that from the station, she walked to the New Panvel side using the sky walk, then she had to cross the highway and there was an HDFC bank branch she would pass. After that, I had heard the sounds of namaz a couple of times in the background as we talked, which meant that there was a mosque somewhere close to her house. Was this information really enough to hunt her down, I wondered. I decided against it, and rang up my friends instead and invited them over to my place, hoping that they would at least divert my mind.

'Huh!' Subho sighed, 'It does seems quite complex.'

Ali and Pritam had also come; I told them about my waking-up-in-the-middle-of-the-night episode.

'What do I do now?' I asked.

'Well, let me think,' said Subho as he strolled lazily towards the balcony. I waited for his expert advice with bated breath.

'Wow! Your society has a big swimming pool!' he yelled out, pointing to the pool below. Sometimes, he was just impossible. My world had always fascinated him for some reason, and so now that he was in my apartment, he and the others hadn't stopped exploring every nook and corner in amazement. No doubt, it was a marvellously done up place; after all, Dad had invested crores to do up his son's bachelor pad. I was amused every time they discovered something that caught their interest. They hadn't yet seen the Jacuzzi in the bathroom.

'Guys! You're here for a reason,' I bawled.

'Yep dude!' Subho replied, 'But can we just take a dip first and then discuss it with a fresh mind?'

I couldn't believe the speed at which Subho then actually ran downstairs, all the way to the pool, with Pritam following him, and how they plunged into the water together. I lit a cigarette and sat on the balcony, watching them swim with the little kids already in the pool. *And these were my mature friends!*

'You said she has a boyfriend,' Ali said, passing me the cigarette after a puff. He wasn't really interested in the matter but somehow, men always tend to talk about something while smoking, and that something is usually either career or women because these are the two reasons why men opt to smoke in the first place.

'Yeah! She did...but they kinda broke up recently.'

'How long did it last?'

'Four years maybe…I am not sure, but that guy was just a jerk.'

'Whatever,' he snubbed.

'I mean he beat her a few times.' I wanted him to know the details even though I knew neither could he do anything about it nor was he interested.

'That's not the point, my friend.'

'Then?'

'Whom do you love? Your Riya or this Ananya?'

'Of course Riya!' The answer came out in a flash.

'That's good then. Fuck this chick, Ananya!'

'Would you please explain what you mean?' I was shocked at his words.

'You're the rebound guy!'

'Now what's that?'

'It's what she thinks of you. She is just playing around.'

'C'mon, she is a nice girl and a very good friend.'

'Woman, not girl. She is twenty-eight. She is very smart. Just look at yourself, if she really thinks of you as a friend then why did she propose to you?'

'She didn't propose. Umm…she just asked me,' I mumbled.

'And my question is why?'

'May be she wants to clear…'

'Clear what? Dude! Don't make a fool of yourself as she is doing to you. Girls are like that, they always want someone around. And you're just an easy guy. And the very simple explanation to this is the four-year difference. She very well knows that nothing could happen between both of you and still she asked you that. She has a boyfriend but she hangs out with you all time. She is using you and you're still not getting it.'

'Phew! Where did all this come from? Which book or movie?' I laughed.

'Yeah! It's really hard for you to digest but it's the truth. Just think about it, did she call you even once afterwards?'

I shook my head. 'She must be busy with her family.'

'So what? You too are with your friends, aren't you thinking of her? She didn't call because she doesn't need you now. See, it's a game with rules, you have to learn the rules and rule the game.'

'Hmmmm,' I sighed and lit the last cigarette.

'Like you love your Riya, she too loves her boyfriend, but he is not around now. She needs you to fill the gap. Talk to her, hang around with her or take her to bed, just be cool about it until you find someone better. They are all the same; they all want the same thing. I mean if not her, you've still got other options around you. Like Mudrika and even Richa, if you can consider her,' he just went on and on, flashing his tobacco stained teeth, laughing at what he thought was a joke. I hoped my deadpan gaze conveyed to him though that the next time he talked like that, he would have to live out the rest of his days drinking his food through a straw.

∽

Over the next two days, Ananya didn't call me even once, nor did she send any message. Back at work on Monday, she did not turn up for our usual post-lunch afternoon walk. I assumed she wouldn't meet me in the evening at the station either. I wasn't upset; for once, I was furious. Was Ali right in everything he had said about her? How could she do this to me, my mind screamed in anguish. Then just when I thought that everything between us had ended, the phone on my table rang, giving me hope. Ananya was calling.

'Ananya! What's wrong with you girl? Where were you these two days?' I couldn't help raising my voice.

'Nothing re! I was just busy,' she said grimly.

'Fine, but why didn't you call me even once?'

'I was busy.'

'Why didn't you come for a walk today?'

'I was really busy.'

No matter what my question, she had the same reply: *I was busy.* So I gave up and came straight to the point.

'Why did you call now? What do you want?'

'What do you mean by that?' She was taken aback. There was a pause; maybe she was waiting for me to say something first but I chose to wait for her instead.

'See, I am trying to open my Gmail account, but it's saying that this site is not trusted.'

Stupid girl! Her BIOS chip was down, I guessed. All she needed to do was reset the date and time and the problem would have been solved. But let her figure it out, I decided.

'I don't know, that's not my job or concern, you should contact the IT system team.'

'OK!' She was stumped.

'Yep! Bye,' and I put the receiver down abruptly.

She called me back.

'Yes?' I answered.

'Why are you so rude today? What's wrong?'

'Nothing, talk to you later. I'm *busy*,' I said and hung up again. And this time I put the receiver off the hook.

∽

As expected, she didn't send me any message while leaving from office nor did I bother doing so. Instead, I made a plan to take my friends out to JavaGreen for coffee. What was the occasion? They did not dare to ask. I just wanted to miss my regular train. Also, I suddenly felt a pang of guilt; these were, in fact, the people who really cared for me and I needed to acknowledge them for that more often. Or so I told myself.

At the coffee shop, the party didn't even begin. Everyone just sat there, passing the menu around to each other, and finally, it came to Subho, who didn't even know the difference between coffee and tea. He simply ordered cold coffee for all of us. When our coffees were served, some of them were looking idly around the café, some were busy checking their cell phones and Pritam seemed to learning the menu card by rote. The usual fun and coziness between us was missing. I was upset, they all knew why and still didn't think of initiating any conversation. We finished our drinks silently, bid each other formal byes and went our separate ways.

Walking back through the campus, I felt low, brooding over all that was happening in my life. Not again, I thought. I had already enough of this feeling when Riya left me and it took me such a lot of time to overcome it. I still hadn't moved on. I was waiting for her to come back someday. But at least I had started smiling again in life. All thanks to my new friends. And yet I behaved so badly with them. Not a big deal though, I would take them out again and things would get better, I consoled myself. Moreover, I felt that I had done the right thing by missing the train. *What gave Ananya the right to treat me the way she did? Who did she think she was? The hell with her. I simply don't care.* And so I went on and on in my head, making my way steadily to the station, listening to Alizee's new number on my headphones. No hurry, no worry and no tension, life really *is* that simple without girls, I decided.

It wasn't that easy though. I reached the station and froze, my mind and my body went numb. Ananya was right there, sitting on our regular bench, reading a book. I wondered what to do, whether I should ignore her or hide or run back the way I came!

'Hey, Gauti!' she greeted.

'Hello,' I said coldly.

Her smile vanished. 'It seems that you weren't expecting me!'

'Nothing like that! What makes you so late today?'

'Since you have waited for me many times earlier, I thought I'd do it for you today.'

'Hmmm,' I grunted.

'What's wrong with you today?'

'Nothing. You tell me, what's new with you.'

'See Gauti, I said I was busy with my family.'

'Did I really ask you anything about that? Your life, your wish. Do whatever you want.'

'I'm sorry.'

'For what?'

'I don't know, Gauti! But you're the only friend I have and don't want to lose you.' I could see a glint of tears near her lashes but I wasn't impressed. Girls could do that at will I knew. I thought instead about how true Ali had been about her and I was determined not to let her get away that easily. The game was on and I made my next move.

'Don't talk like that, Anu, I'm always there for you, because I...' I paused intentionally. Sometimes, even the unsaid words conveyed the right message. It was all about manipulation with the right special effects, you see.

'Because I...I mean you...complete what you want to say.'

'Of course...I love you.'

Till I find someone better.

Anything for You, Ma'am!

I was pissed off responding to Muthu's pings asking for the status every half hour, so after a while, I just ignored his messages. I was aware that this would annoy him, especially after that portal episode. He never said that I had done a good job; instead was always caustic when I made a mistake. He never thought it necessary to instruct me on what to do or why. What did he think, I was telepathic? He played his subordinates against each other and then chuckled as they clashed. He kept favourites and coddled them, bullying anyone who crossed his path. He even took credit for work that I had done and lied about his contribution. He expected me to be on call all the time, ruining my evenings and weekends. Yet he bad-mouthed me to higher-ups and I could not even counter him because he would do it all privately. He badly needed to learn some managerial skills himself, but would never acknowledge it of course. Emotionally unstable and corrupt, he openly encouraged a culture of corruption at work.

There...I guess I had enough reason to call him a pig.

Yet another ping! But this time, it was a message from Subho: *Lunch?*

An idle mind is the devil's workshop and I had worked very hard in this workshop. I stood up and stretched lazily, yawning loud enough for all to hear how dedicated I was to my job.

'Deshmukh!' Muthu shouted out at my retreating back. 'Status?'

'Yeah! Sir, I did run the tool and found a few minor bugs right at the start. I'm correcting them. I mean, sending them to the vendors will actually take a lot of time, so I thought...'

'Who told you to think?' he interrupted me. 'You are here to test tools and not to think,' he barked, displaying this great knack he had at insulting people. *Bastard,* I muttered under my breath. 'OK, I will complete it after lunch,' I gave in.

'No, you're completing it now.'

Pig! Pig! Pig! My soul screamed as I went back to my desk.

'You know you're just trying too hard. Nothing's gonna help you,' Ali offered.

'Maybe you're right, I need to try something else.'

'Like what?'

'Don't know yet but to make the deaf hear, you need to try an explosion.'

'Huh! Dude, you sound scary. All the best for your explosion,' he smiled.

❧

'I need to tell you something,' Ananya initiated rather anxiously, on our regular post-lunch walk that day.

'Tell me.' I had already sensed something fishy in her unusually quiet behaviour.

'I hope you won't get angry.'

I shook my head but I was already fuming within. First, Muthu had spoiled my mood and now Ananya was getting there.

'Well…Sachin called me yesterday.'

'What's the big deal in that? He calls you every day.'

'No. I mean, tomorrow is 4th December.'

'So?'

'It's our fourth anniversary. We met first on this very day.'

'Hmmm.'

'See, he wants me to go out with him,' she paused to see my reaction and I gave her what she wanted, a stern gaze.

'Just for the last time, he said. He wants to end it on a good note.'

'So, you want my permission?'

For some time, she remained silent and when we reached her block, I stopped.

'Bye,' I said curtly and turned to walk towards my block.

'Gauti! Wait,' she called.

I turned to her.

'How rude is that? You're leaving a lady like that,' she complained.

'What?' I was baffled. 'Let me clarify for you, I do this every day. If you ever cared to turn and look back, you'd know.'

'Gauti!' She walked the distance between us and came so close that her hair blowing with the breeze touched my cheeks. It looked like we were to kiss and I wouldn't have minded that, even if it cost me my job for misconduct on campus.

'You said you love me,' she pestered.

'So?' I countered, 'Does it matter to you? You never said that to me.'

She frowned, 'I'll say that when the right time comes.'

'Hmmm.' I was bored of listening to that theory.

'Gauti, say something.'

'OK! Fine. Go with him, I don't mind. Seriously.'

'That's it?' She raised her eyebrow.

'What else do you expect?'

'OK! Whatever. Bye.' She abruptly turned around and walked back to her block.

Back at my desk, Muthu gave me a dirty look from where he sat; it was fifteen minutes past the end of my lunch break. I had already completed my work for the day but didn't tell Muthu about it lest he assigned me something else. So instead, I sat chatting with my friends on Facebook. It wouldn't take a genius to guess whom I would kill if I was legally allowed one murder!

'Hello!' Ananya had called.

'Yes?'

'You busy?'

'Ya, kind of.'

'I'm sorry for today.'

'Anu it's OK! Please. I have some work now.'

'Just called to tell you that I'm not going.'

'And why so?'

'He asked me to reach Panvel at 7 and that's impossible if I leave after 6.'

Only girls could be so obtuse, was she really expecting me to give her a solution?

'C'mon, he can wait for you for some time.'

'You're taunting me. Just chuck the idea, forget it.'

'Listen Anu, I don't know what to say about it but I want you to go. I mean c'mon, you guys were together for years, so a last date is a really good idea.'

'I wonder what you mean by that. Anyway, I told you, I would miss the 6.07 train and reach late, he wouldn't understand and then we would fight.'

'See, Anu. Leave that to me. I'll handle that.'

There was a big and crazy idea brewing in my mind and I knew it was really risky. But this was the only way to get noticed, I felt. I simply couldn't waste all my days searching for bugs. However, I knew I couldn't do it alone and needed a helping hand. Which was kinda impossible since the consequences could cost us our jobs or land us in jail. But I knew there was one other maniac like me who would understand.

'You've simply gone out of your mind. It's not that simple to break into the company's firewall. They will come to know immediately and the security will detain us in less than a minute.' Ali protested vehemently when I told him about the plan.

'Yeah that's what I want. I want to tell them that if a guy can break into their security so easily, then he is capable of doing far more than this testing crap.'

'Still…'

'We are just going to change the time shown in the company network; we aren't hacking any information. It's just to prove our potential.'

'They will throw us out.'

'Oh c'mon Ali! If you're worrying about this fucking job, I'll get you something better with my dad's contacts.'

'OK,' he said half heartedly. 'But there is one condition.'

'What?'

'Get me a whole crate of imported cigars,' Ali demanded.

Phew! I thought he would ask me for a date.

'Deal.'

We shook hands.

∽

'I can't believe I'm actually helping you in this,' Ali said as both of us eased into the server room. He stood as a cover at the door while I sat to work on our department's server.

The first step was to unlock the server which was accessible only to the admin. Pritam and I had just three chances to guess the password. I thought for a while about the possibilities and a very old logic came to my mind. I typed a possible password and pressed Enter. Bingo! On the first attempt. Half the job was done, now I only had to break into the company firewall, access the network, search for the system that maintained the centralized company clock, hack it and forward the time by ten minutes.

I called Ananya 'Hey! Get ready.'

'But there's still some time for six.'

'It will be time to leave in another moment, you better pack your stuff.'

'What's happening Gautam?' I could sense panic in her voice.

'Nothing. You wanted to leave before six, right?'

'Hmm…' she grunted.

'So…anything for you, Ma'am.'

I don't know whether I was expecting a thank you or whether she was feeling guilty, but both of us were silent for a moment. Was she breathing heavily because she shared my awkwardness or was she nervous about the evening ahead? Of course, it wasn't their first date, but then, things between them were not creating sparks anymore. Also, now I was somewhere in the picture. I consoled myself that letting her go with him implied that she meant nothing to me. *I just want to sleep with her*, I told myself.

'Anu! Just enjoy the evening. Good bye,' I said casually and hung up.

Five minutes of typing, a bit of logic and my all knowledge from engineering let me in through the firewall. As I hit the main server, Ali watched anxiously, standing behind me. Every time I missed something, I would turn to him for help and his super brain would have already calculated the escape route. And with the final Enter, I heard a long beep sound across all the security locks, and then came the dialogue box that notified me that the operation was successful.

It was six o' clock all over the company, ten minutes before the actual hour.

I gave Ali a high five, 'We did it.'

'Yay! We...we did it,' Ali stammered. We had committed the sin and now waited for redemption.

Within a minute, the intrusion was noticed and traced. Realizing the gravity of our act, I wanted Ali to get out of the room. After all, it had been my crazy idea and I didn't want him to get into trouble. But the pretty smile on his face meant that he too didn't care about the consequences anymore. Yes! We did it and we wanted to tell everyone. We waited inside the server room for security guards. The big buzzer ringing outside had created panic on the floor and people were gathering around, looking clueless and asking each other what was happening.

Five, four, three, two, one...Knock! Knock! BUSTED.

⚮

'You are both fired from your job with immediate effect!' That was our HR head.

The big disco was attended by many high officials, including the CEO of the company and our HOD Mr Bose. While the rest of the crowd kept blabbering all kinds of allegations and arguing about the penalty, Mr Bose just stood staring at us. He was more upset than angry; we looked down to avoid his eyes, because the truth was that we had done something really wrong.

'Ask the security to beat them black and blue.' 'Call the police and throw them in jail.' 'Mark them in the blacklist so that they never get jobs anywhere.'

'Just tell me why you did this?' Mr Bose asked us quietly.

We didn't even dare look at him, let alone come up with an answer.

'I want to know,' he stamped his fist on the conference table and that shook everybody.

'No bad intentions, Sir,' I mumbled.

'Then what?'

No reply.

'This silence won't help, young men. If you don't open your mouth, I will have to seek police help.'

'Ha! Police for what? I'm really apologetic about breaching your security but I still feel that we deserve some appreciation,' Ali spoke confidently.

'I'm sorry...I just can't understand what you mean?' The CEO questioned.

'Which part did you not understand Ma'am?'

'You think you're Mark Zuckerberg?'

'No, I'm not. I have a better hair style,' I smiled. My joke was not taken in the right spirit though and the board gave us disgusted looks.

'We just brought to your notice the holes in the security. I mean, it just took me ten minutes to break into the security.'

'You should have communicated this to your seniors directly.'

'Do you think people would have taken us seriously?'

'Why not?'

'No comments on that. Just want to say that if we guys can hack the security, then I guess we deserve more than this stupid testing job.'

'What do you want?'

'I told you. Some appreciation.'

People stood gaping at each other but I was done proving my point and so was the board with their prosecution, I guessed. The

CEO discussed a few things with her subordinates while we all waited for her decision with bated breath.

'Well, Mr Deshmukh and Mr Ali, we do get your point and are going to discuss the same in this month's board meeting at your presence. Secondly, though I very well understand that you both didn't have bad intentions, but what you did was a crime and cannot be ignored, so disciplinary measures have to be taken. We will take a final call on this and notify you by Monday.'

We nodded in approval.

'Enough for now. I call off the meeting,' she said.

Whether the final verdict would be positive or negative, it didn't matter. Somewhere down the line, it was our personal victory, though of course, no one was congratulating us. Probably because of the CEO's presence or maybe an attitude of professionalism prevented them from coming forward and shaking hands with us. However, the twitching lips on so many faces as they all passed us on their way out said a lot; it gave us our much needed recognition.

'Mr Deshmukh! I am impressed with your confidence and hope things go right for you. Anyway, I really want both of you to be involved in new innovation drives ahead,' the CEO said as she walked past us in the lobby.

'Anything for you, Ma'am,' we said in chorus.

Trust Me

We were suspended from work for three days and following that was a weekend, so that basically meant a five-day holiday for Ali and me in Alibaug, where we survived largely on alcohol and cigarettes. When we returned, we were given a grand welcome. Our security hacking heroics had made us small-time celebrities on campus. The news had spread everywhere. We found people recognizing us, smiling at us or talking about us when we passed by. The BPO girls hovered near our table, giggling and gossiping in the food court.

Subho labelled us The Geek Studs. Gosh! He was so jealous of all the attention we were getting.

'You know what, this is not going to last for long,' he said.

'So what? Why do you think I care?' I replied.

He couldn't think of any smart response, so he popped a spoonful of fried rice in his mouth instead and avoided looking at me after that. I knew my answer had hurt him. But I always enjoyed piercing his inflated ego.

'It happens Subho. As they say, success is hard to digest. Not your own but your friends' success,' I taunted him some more.

'Listen dude! I know what success is. I'm a published author, remember?' he tried another tack.

I had planned my response to that long ago.

'Whether you're a published author or a porn star, who the fuck cares? Let me enjoy my piece of cake too.' I had always wanted to tell him this to his face and I did. Yippee!

He was shocked and dumbfounded at that. The expression on his face was worth capturing on camera, so I quickly tried retrieving my phone from my pocket but before I could, Subho stormed out of the place in disgust. And I loved it.

After lunch, I called Ananya out for a walk; I hadn't heard from her since her anniversary date. She had called a few times while I was in Alibaug but I had been so sloshed, I couldn't even crawl to the table to pick up the phone. She seemed more concerned than excited when I met her outside her block. Both of us had a lot to catch up. We smiled as our eyes met and set out on our familiar route.

'Where were you?' she asked.

'Out for a holiday,' I beamed.

'Hmm. Had a great time then?'

I grunted, 'As if you didn't have fun here?'

She glared at me.

'What? Why you're looking at me like that? I mean, you went out with him that evening.'

'So?'

'Nothing. I understand that it's something personal and you don't want to share. Fine.'

She seemed subdued and looked away. Unlike her usual habit, she didn't crush the dry leaves scattered all around as she walked nor did she hum old melodies. She seemed lost in her own world. Whatever was bothering her, I wanted her to tell me about it without my asking. So I also remained silent and that only hurt her more. Now and then she looked at me imploringly, prompting me with her eyes to ask her something, but I pretended not to notice.

'You didn't call me even once?' she finally broke the silence.

'Well, I told you I was out. I was in Alibaug with my friends and I forgot to take my cell with me.' I lied so that I would not need to justify ignoring her calls.

'When did you leave?'

'On Wednesday.'

'Why didn't you call on Tuesday then?'

'Are you mad?' I reacted instantly. 'You were out with your Sachin, celebrating your anniversary, so do you think I would've disturbed you?'

'Oh! Shut up. Just shut up,' she sobbed.

'What happened?'

'Nothing. Just leave it.' And with that, the tears came pouring down her cheeks. I made her sit down on a bench.

'It's OK Anu. What's wrong? Tell me,' I tried consoling her. She tugged at my shoulder and pulled me towards her. Next thing I know, she was in my arms, weeping aloud. I looked around in apprehension. Luckily there wasn't anybody around. But you never knew who was watching you, what with so many CCTV cameras installed all over the campus. But hey, who could really push a girl like Ananya away? I held her even more tightly.

'Anu! Don't cry like this. What's the matter, please tell me?'

'Nothing,' she said, still crying.

'C'mon tell me.'

'Sachin didn't turn up at all that evening. I waited for three hours but he was nowhere to be seen.'

'You should have called him on his cell then.'

'I did. But it was switched off,' she mumbled through her tears. She hugged me even tighter then and suddenly, it wasn't casual anymore. I had goose bumps all over.

'Control yourself, Anu. We're still on campus,' I said to her.

'Yeah!' she grunted and pushed me away. She wiped her tears and said, 'I need to go.' And just like that, she walked away, leaving me behind on the bench. Was I supposed to stop her? Maybe, but I didn't. I watched her disappear behind the BPO block and walked back to my own block, listening to Phil Collins sing *Against all odds* on my iPod.

✒

'I think this is the best chance you have,' Ali said when I had told him everything that had happened. 'Call her now.'

'Nah! She is upset,' I shook my head.

'That's why I'm saying, ask her for a date. She won't say no. And then, I guess I need not tell you what to do,' he ended with a wink.

'Date? Where should I take her? Movie? Beach? Restaurant?'

'Let me think…Umm…Karnala!'

'Now what's that?'

'Hey! It's a bird sanctuary on the Alibaug road.'

'Are you mad? That's a bloody jungle,' I protested.

'That's simply the best. Trust me!'

'And how do you think I'll convince her?'

'Now that's up to you. Let's see your talent. Anyway, if she agrees to come, then she is all yours.'

I could only nod in reply to that.

'Call her now!' he ordered.

'No. I'll talk to her about this in the train.'

∽

She had sent me a couple of messages, but they were forwarded ones, reminding me to call and comfort a friend in time of need, and so on. But I had by then learnt how to dominate the game. So naturally, I didn't call or send any message.

'Hi!' She greeted me when we met at the station.

I gave her a small smile.

'I'm sorry.'

'For what?'

'I left you alone on the bench.'

'You always do that.'

'I was upset.' She paused for a moment and broke down again. 'He didn't come. It was our anniversary.'

'So was it my fault?'

'No,' she shook her head. 'I'm sorry.'

'Not again Anu. Get into the train first.'

I had to somehow bring up the idea of the date but didn't know how to begin. I was scared of what her reaction would be. I mean, Karnala sounded really bizarre even to me, but it was a challenge. I had to go for it and had even thought of a possible way of convincing her. But two stations went by and I had still not uttered a word.

'What's that you're murmuring?' she caught me.

'Nothing,' I said sheepishly.

'What is it?' she demanded and smiled just a little bit, 'Say it.'

'Well…I was thinking…maybe we could go out somewhere?'

'Meaning?'

'I mean, I know how you felt when he didn't turn up, so I thought I'd cheer you up.'

'Hmm…but where?'

'Karnala fort?'

'What?!'

'Oh it's a nice place. It has a historical dimension too. And a trekking adventure, beautiful natural surroundings, wildlife and all. It would be fun, what say?' I went on to narrate all the positives I could think of that a place like Karnala would offer, hoping she wouldn't smell the real kill.

'Sounds cool. I need to think about it.'

'Trust me Anu. You're gonna love this.'

'OK!' And she changed the subject.

❧

'She agreed,' I told Ali on the phone later.

'That's great, Tiger!' he congratulated. 'By the way, did she say yes or OK?'

'What?'

'Did she say the word yes or OK?'

'What's the difference?'

'Yes or OK?'

'OK.'

'Well then…*Dilli abhi door hai bhai.*'

I don't know what he reckoned from that 'OK', but he didn't say anything more. I figured I needed to put in some more effort and coax Ananya sweetly. I later realized that was actually a big mistake and that was how I lost control over the game. I became extra caring to her, increased the frequency of my calls and messages, complimented her with e-cards, downloaded her favourite songs, and even went to the temple with her, twice. Whenever we met, I talked excitedly about the D-day and praised Karnala as if it were the mystic Kashmir. But still, it was always only an 'OK' I got from her.

∽

'Hello! Hello! Anu! You there?' I kept screaming while she stayed mum on the other side.

'Ya…' she sighed.

'What happened?' I was nervous, I knew that something was fishy.

'I got my medical reports.'

'What do they say?' Sweat trickled down my brow, I wondered what was coming.

'I'm pregnant,' she sobbed.

'What???' I was shell-shocked to hear those two words. 'Are you sure about it?'

'What do you mean by that? Karnala was your idea only na?' she bawled.

She continued to curse me while that P-word almost gave me a mini heart attack. The receiver fell from my hand and my feet were trembling. I sat like a statue with all my senses blanked out and my whole body gone cold. My heart was pounding hard as if I had just run a marathon. I assumed my brain was dead; there was no response at all as I kept myself asking what next.

'Hey, Gauti. What's up? Are you okay?' Subho asked me. I nodded weakly. Somehow I could not find my voice.

'It's not OK! What's the matter?' Richa joined in. Seated close to me, I was sure she had overheard my conversation with Ananya.

'Let's go outside!' I pleaded to Subho.

We walked out to the smoking area. Ali lit a cigarette and passed it to me. I took a long puff as if to burn it down in a single breath and let out a cloud of smoke, coughing hard. The nicotine hit my blocked brain and did its bit. I immediately felt light-headed and leaned against the wall.

'See, dude! We are not here to see your smoking feat. Tell us what's the matter,' Richa said as she snatched the cigarette and took a puff. She was way ahead of us here too, she could make smoke rings.

I told them everything and going by their expression, I reckoned the situation was beyond their worst nightmares. All of them began abusing me. Richa even slapped me.

'How could you do this? Damn! What will I say to my dad if he comes to know that my friends have sex before marriage?' That was Moody of course.

'Moody shut up!' I yelled.

Richa slapped me again.

'Whose idea was Karnala?' Subho asked.

'Ali suggested it,' I pointed to Ali.

'I did tell you to take her there but didn't tell you to get her pregnant,' Ali defended himself.

'Whatever. Couldn't you get a condom? Moron! How could you be so careless?' Richa was furious.

'What will you do now, Gauti? Abortion?!' Ali answered.

'Are you mad? You will kill little Chintu?' Moody shrieked.

'Now who is this Chintu?!' I thought I was going mad.

'Your kid!'

'Oh God! People please take her out of my sight before I kill her.'

I wondered what was funny because everyone was in splits after that. And here I was worrying about how Didi wouldn't talk to me, Mom would cry and Dad would throw me out of the house. I would have to get married to Ananya, there was no other option. I would have to continue working under Muthu for the rest of my life to support my family. I would sing my kid lullabies and change diapers in the middle of night. I would feed my kid, wash his clothes, take him to school and at night, do his homework. I knew my life was ruined; I would grow old and weak under this burden. I would tan, my skin would wrinkle. I would lose all my hair and get a pot-belly.

'No! No!' I screamed in despair.

'Gautam Baba! Gautam Baba! What happened? Wake up!'

'What? What?' I opened my eyes and sat up. Kantabai was shaking me by the shoulder. Gosh! It was just a bad dream then! I sighed in relief. I reached out for my cell. There was a message from Ananya which I ignored; I first wanted to check what day it was. So it was Friday, we hadn't gone anywhere yet. I opened her message, her regular *suprabhat seva*.

I was late that morning and missed our regular train, so I couldn't meet her. I bought a newspaper but other than the title *Mumbai Mirror*, I couldn't read a word. I flipped through the pages, last night's nightmare still haunting my mind and giving me cold shivers. Maybe I should just drop this idea of Karnala, to hell with Ali's challenge, I thought. To divert my mind, I turned to the sports page but an article in the health section caught my attention.

'Give me a packet of condoms,' I asked the chemist outside the station.

Myths you need to know the first time you have sex was the article headline.

∽

'Big day tomorrow, all the best!' Ali gave me a high-five as I left for the station that evening. I quietly slipped out of the office to avoid curious looks from others; Ali had been doing quite a publicity stunt all day.

Ananya met me directly at the station that day. Of course, I already knew that something was wrong but the excitement of the next day was topmost in my mind. I walked to the station humming to the tunes of Dr Zeus on my iPod.

'Hi!' I waved to her from a distance and she gave me a tiny smile.

'How was your day?' I asked.

She shrugged and walked towards to the ladies compartment of the train. I reached out for her hand. She glared at me and let go of my hand. She continued listening to music, avoiding my eyes. We boarded the train and sat opposite each other.

'Are you going to talk today?' I was baffled.

'I'm sorry. This track is just awesome!' she said. I took one earplug and listened for about two seconds, then threw it back on her lap.

'Himesh?! Yuck.'

'You are so rude!'

'And what about you?'

'Wait,' she said as her phone began ringing. 'Ma is doing well. I'll get that checkup done…' And her conversation went on for a while although I suspected that she was prolonging it just so that I would hear about her family issues. I plugged in my earphones again.

The train reached Panvel and she finally hung up. I had waited all that time to talk about the outing but she simply walked off ahead without even saying a proper goodbye.

'Ananya!' I called after her again and again. She turned around on my third attempt. She gave me a look that said *What*?!

'Karnala?'

'I will call you.'

'No. Now!' I demanded.

She was silent for a moment. 'I can't commit now. I have some stuff to do tomorrow.'

'Yes or no.'

'Gauti! You must have heard, I was talking to the doctor and will have to take Mom for a check-up.'

'We planned this a week ago. Then how come you take an appointment now?'

'It was an emergency.'

'Yeah I know how urgent it is. You should have just told me a no. Why this drama?'

'What? How can you think so selfishly?' she yelled and turned away.

'Is it me? Damn it! You are selfish,' I replied. 'You just need me when you're down. You don't care one bit for me. For me, you may be my little piece of sunshine but for you, I'm a bucket full of shit.'

'And what do you want? As if I don't know anything. I have seen four summers more than you. It's just that you want to take this girl to bed and that's why you are being so nice to me.'

I was stunned, as if lightening had struck me. I didn't know whether I should defend myself or argue back. She walked away into the crowd. Calling out her name wouldn't have helped. I didn't want to create a scene. I waited for the crowd to disperse but she was gone. I tried her number many times but she didn't pick up. Ultimately, I sent her a message saying I'm sorry and returned home.

She didn't reply.

Three Makes a Crowd

*W*asn't her behaviour the previous evening enough of a hint that she didn't want to come? Yet I waited for her to call or to at least send me a message. And of course, she didn't. I don't know when I slept, but when I woke up, the rays of the evening sun were streaming in through the windows. By the time, I finally got to my feet, it was almost dark. *No use now, Karnala park would have closed for the day,* I laughed to myself and lit a cigarette.

I decided to take my little Beetle out for a ride. I drove all the way to Bandra without taking my foot off the accelerator even once until I reached my destination. An average nightclub on the fringes of a posh locality, I decided to spend the rest of the night there to drink till I rolled on the ground and made up some sort of story for Ali.

'Hey! Give me another. This time make it neat.' A guy sitting next to me at the bar demanded.

'Sir! You've already drunk a lot. I can't serve you anymore,' the bartender refused politely.

'Peene do abhi shaam baki hai,
Abhi unke naam ka ek aur jaam baki hai,
Jana hai maikhane se aaj ladkhadate hue,
Peene do abhi kadmo main thodi jaan baaki hai.'

He was spouting poetry.

'Sorry Sir! No,' the bartender shook his head firmly.

'How dare you refuse me? You know who I am?' The man got aggressive.

'No sir. It doesn't matter, I can't serve you anymore.'

'You bloody asshole!' he screamed and held the bartender by

his collar. The poor chap yelled for help and two bouncers came running instantly. A big drama was to follow. One bouncer grabbed his shoulder and pulled him by the neck while the other tried to drag him away holding on to his waist. The drunk guy tightened his grip but his loud growl was lost in the earsplitting rock music playing in the background. As a last resort, one of the bouncers kicked him in the groin and the guy gave in. He fell on the ground, moaning in pain. Together, the bouncers picked him up and dealt a few slaps to his face. They dragged him out. My eyes followed him through. And when he stood swaying under the lights near the door, I could finally see his face.

He was tall and lanky. He was very dark, black I would say, and not in the least bit handsome. Perhaps, I would even put his photo alongside 'ugly' in the dictionary to explain the meaning of the word perfectly. His bushy coconut-oiled hair made him look even more terrible. Seriously, if I had a face like his, I would have sued my parents. The bouncers kicked him out.

'*Ladki kutty cheez hai,*' the bartender sighed.

Gosh! Even a guy as ugly as that had a girlfriend and here I was craving for love and burning myself. Where was the fairness in this world!

She hadn't called me yet. I finished another drink and decided I had had enough for the day. I had to drive back home, I had to go to office the next day. Such was my life! When I had passed out of college, I remember how free I had felt. I was the king lion, I would roar and the world would fear me. But in the end, I became a dog, a dog to a pig like Muthu. I sighed aloud.

I had just driven a couple of streets when the same nightclub guy caught my attention. He was strolling groggily along the footpath. It was too late in the night and for the sake of humanity, I wanted to help him. So I honked a couple of times to catch his attention but it only irked him.

'Fuck off! You motherfucker,' he shouted. I contemplated kicking his face.

Ladki kutty cheez hai. The line rankled in my head and that very line saved him. I understood his pain. And anyway, why should I improve his looks by breaking a few of his teeth, I asked myself.

'Buddy! Take it easy. I want to help,' I said.

'Why? Who are you? What do you want?'

'I was sitting next to you in the club. It's very late. I'll drop you to your place.'

'No. Go away. Leave me alone.'

To hell with him then. To hell with humanity. I got back into my car but before speeding away, I gave it a last try. I stepped hard on the accelerator and my little pet thundered like a tiger.

'*Dost!* Please wait,' he called. This act always works, I smiled. I opened the door.

'Nice car you have!' He complimented me and relaxed in the seat.

I nodded and smiled.

'Where do you want to go?' I asked.

'*Jaana toh bahut door hai, bas manzil ka pata nahi*!' he mumbled and laughed. I gave him a cold stare. He had a French beard that was only visible up close. The piercings over his eyebrows and earlobes and tattoos everywhere only confirmed how much he hated being himself. The scars and scratches on his face meant that he often had a face-off with such bouncers. Moreover, he kept trying out all the buttons in my baby and fiddled with everything within his reach. Those one liners simply pissed me off. I regretted giving him the lift. His presence suffocated me. I seriously considered kicking him out mid-way.

'Here is the bus stop, you can go anywhere you want,' I stopped my car.

He gave me a stern look, raising his eyebrows. 'You said you will drop me at my place.'

'Then for god's sake tell me where you want to go,' I said.

He smiled. 'Who is she?'

'What?'

'You gave me a lift because you could relate to my story. You pitied me because you see yourself in me,' he said. *I saw myself in him? Bullshit! He looks like the dog in the Vodafone ads*, I thought.

'So?' he grunted.

I shook my head.

'You can tell me,' he insisted. *Who did he think he was? Shahrukh Khan?* And anyway, what should I have told him? Riya, a girl who thought I was a loser in life, had dumped me. So I had come to Mumbai, leaving behind my dad's big business, to lick Muthu's ass just to prove a point to Riya. And Ananya? I wanted to sleep with her because she looked like Riya, but again, she turned out to be smarter than me.

'Whatever!' he gave up. 'I love my girl.'

'Hmmm.'

'But she thinks I'm a loser.' *Yeah. All girls are the same.*

'It's OK, buddy!' I patted his back. 'I understand. Do you both talk?'

'No. Very rare.'

'You still love her?'

He nodded.

'Then call her and tell her that you love her.' I know that wasn't great advice or anything new that I was telling him but I couldn't think of anything else then.

He smiled and dialled a number.

'Damn!' he frowned, 'It's busy.'

'Is it?' I comforted, 'Try again.'

'Ya,' he grunted. 'I guess your phone is ringing.'

'What?' I checked the back seat; my phone was dancing to the tune of Bombay Rockers. I checked the screen. *Ananya calling.*

'Buddy you keep trying, I'll just attend this call,' I excused myself and got out of the car.

'Hello Ananya!' I answered.

'Hi Gauti!' she greeted, 'What's up?'

'Nothing.'

'I'm sorry that I ditched you today. But please understand me, I need some time.'

'Hmm…'

'By the way, where are you?'

'I'm out.'

'I know what you mean by that. You must be boozing around somewhere.'

'Not like that, Ananya.'

'I'm sorry; I know you're drinking because of me.'

'Forget it!' I cut in. 'How was your day? How was Auntie's checkup?'

And it went on and on for the next half hour. I completely forgot that I had a jerk inside my car. Finally, my phone battery begged me to cut the call.

'Oops! Ananya! My battery is low. Need to hang up.'

'That's not fair, I'm not finished yet.'

'I know! I will call you once I reach home,' I got into the car and saw the ugly snob fiddling with the music player. He gave me a look as if I was his paid driver but I was in a good mood by then.

'Sorry dude! Was on a call till now.'

'Gauti! Who is with you?'

'A guy.'

'You're a gay?'

'Bye,' I cut the call.

'Your girl?' he asked. *Was she?*

I nodded and asked him, 'You talked to yours?'

'Nah! Her number was busy all the while.'

'Must be some bastard. Find him and kick his ass.'

∞

Always have a smile on your face in the mornings, it keeps people curious and imaginative about your stints of the previous night. And that's what I did to Ali. He was dying for some gossip but was too obstinate to ask me about it directly. I did a pretty good job of blushing.

Slowly things between me and Ananya started to improve. Autumn was back again. Long calls, SMS chats, train travel, afternoon walks and even lunch together sometimes. I thought a few times about giving Ali's challenge a second try but I wanted to go easy and not repeat my mistakes. *Let's give it some more time as Ananya says*, I thought.

My phone screen flashed *Ananya calling*. Time to leave the office.

'Hello Anu! I'm just packing, will be outside your block in two minutes,' I said, gathering my things.

'No, Gauti! Go ahead. I'll be late today. There's some work here.'

'OK then! Don't worry, Ma'am. You complete your work, I'll wait for you.'

'What? Pathetic you are!' she shouted. 'You're simply getting on my nerves.'

Did I hear right? Why was she reacting like that, I wondered.

'What happened?' I asked.

'Just go away. I don't want to see you anywhere around me. Do you get that?' and she cut the call.

I was bewildered. What was that all about? She could be so weird! Forget about her! *Can't I go home alone*, I said aloud. I had an iPod, a Blackberry phone with high speed internet, Durjoy Datta's latest novel in my bag, and even a business magazine I had picked up from the office library. Was I going to Nerul or was I flying to New York?

And still all that was not enough. I could do nothing but think about Ananya. Her presence was becoming a bad habit but I didn't bother asking myself whether it was lust or love. I called her a few times but her phone was switched off. I sent an SMS and waited for the delivery report. I was worried. I even thought about going over to her office but her words held me back. I waited for her at Nerul station, hoping she would change trains there but I knew that would happen only if she didn't get a direct train. I was ready to take a chance but how long should I wait, I wondered. *Until I get that damn delivery report and then I can call her.*

One hour passed by. The ladies special, two direct Panvel trains, four Nerul trains and numerous other locals went by but I sat unmoving on platform no.1. I glanced at the LED indicator for the umpteenth time. A Panvel fast was to come in ten minutes. She usually took this one but she wouldn't get off the train I knew. I paced the area where the ladies compartment would halt.

Suddenly, I saw her standing at a distance, near the gate of the station. I could recognize that green salwar anywhere. But why would she stand there, I wondered. That was where the general compartment halted. I walked ahead and a few steps later, I knew it was definitely my Ananya. I broke into a jog but she noticed me only when I nearly crashed into her. The little smile on her face vanished instantly as our eyes met.

'Hi, Anu!' I said.

'Gauti!' she froze. 'What are you doing here?'

'It's a railway station, a public place.'

'You've been following me?'

'C'mon Ananya, why would I?'

'Whatever. You need to go now.'

'But why? What's wrong?'

'Ananya!' A hoarse voice called out behind me.

I turned to see a tall and thin black guy was holding a Pepsi bottle in one hand and a plate of samosas in the other. I turned back to Ananya; she looked terrified. *But wait a minute, did I know this guy?* I turned back to look at him properly. Gosh! It was Mr World (in the ugly category) from the other night at the pub. What was he doing with Ananya?

'Gautam, this is Sachin Masane. My boyfriend!' Ananya explained.

My boyfriend? Those two words echoed in my brain. I felt as if the roof of Nerul station had just fallen on my head. I desperately wished that the earth would open up and swallow me. I wanted to jump onto the tracks and wanted the fast train to run over me. It would at least have ended all feeling. I prayed desperately that what I had heard was just a bad joke.

'Sachin, he is Gautam Deshmukh. My colleague,' Ananya introduced me.

'Hi Gautam!' He shook my hand.

'Hello!'

'Have we met before? I mean, your face seems so familiar.'

'Is it? I don't think so,' I quickly denied it.

'That Andheri pub? You're the guy with that expensive car.'

'Car? Expensive? Then it's definitely not him. Sachin, he works in my office.'

'Yeah you see, we are paid peanuts there.' And that wasn't even a joke but the ugly duckling standing in front of me almost fell down laughing. *Yuck! What a bad choice, Ananya!*

'Whatever! I owe a lot to that guy, I got back my love just because of him,' and he planted a kiss on her head and pulled her towards him to give her a tight hug.

This was the last straw. It tore me apart. I turned away. I don't know what Ananya's reaction was; after all, it was a public place. The train came in at that moment and both of them boarded it holding hands. She waved at me but I was already rushing out of the station.

I didn't eat that night. I cried a little and smoked a lot, sitting in the balcony. Ananya called me late at night. I cut her call but she called again. I switched off my phone.

Did I actually think we were in a relationship? I had been losing control all along and her dominating behaviour had just got worse each day. Ali had warned me of the consequences but I had turned a deaf ear. Well, that's what you call the 'hangover' of love or lust. Or another simple word for it was 'stupidity'.

Love, Life and a Beer Can

'Check this out!' Samir threw an envelope onto my desk.
'What's this?' I grunted and quickly opened it. Inside was a brochure advertising a resort. 'Go Goa' was written in big bold letters in the top right corner. It didn't take a second to guess what Samir was up to. 'No way, I simply can't make it. Sorry!'

'C'mon! It will be real fun.'

'You see I have stuff to complete and besides, my parents won't allow me.' I tried to excuse myself.

'Ah! Don't give that parents shit. Don't be childish, give it a thought first.'

'You and me alone?' I asked. Going on a holiday with seniors was the same as accompanying your parents on a pilgrimage.

'Nah! You can ask your friends to join in.'

We had a big discussion over lunch about the Goa trip. Needless to say, Moody shed tears since we couldn't possibly return from Goa before dark. So it was to be an all-boys tour (Richa was never considered a girl). However, Richa lost out in the lottery we had to do in the end, since my car could carry only five of us, although I did think leaving Samir or even Subho behind would have been better. At least Richa never puked after boozing.

'Jingle bell, jingle bell, jingle all the way. Santa Claus is coming to town riding on a sleigh,' Moody had been irritating everyone with her rhyme since morning.

'Will you please shut the fuck up?' I snapped.

'How rude! It's Christmas today.'

'It's tomorrow, dumbo. Today is the twenty-fourth.' But Christmas was celebrated every year in our company on 24th December.

'Whatever. I just can't wait to see Santa Claus. My friend has just messaged me that he's left from their floor. Next stop is ours! Yippee!' she screamed in joy.

'Are you a five-year-old girl? Don't tell me you hung stockings in your childhood?'

'What? I still do, and see, today he is coming.'

'Gosh! He is some Fatso from HR!' Engineers simply hated the HR staff because even after doing no real work other than these stupid activities in the office, they walked away with more respect, honour, and most importantly, a better package.

'Shut up! You won't understand. Look, he is here. Yayy!' She ran to the door.

'Ouuuch!' I screamed, she had stamped my foot in her hurry. I looked at the lobby. Mr Santa was singing while two other bitches from HR dressed as Santa helpers danced around him, tinkling bells in their hands.

People gathered around them as Santa heaved his big sack from his shoulders and took out chocolates. People mobbed him like they were victims from Haiti waiting for food supplies.

'This is for you, cute little girl,' Santa gave a handful of chocolates to Moody.

'This for you, Mr Expressionless,' he turned to me.

'What just one chocolate for me? You gave her so many,' I argued.

'Hah!' he laughed and went ahead.

'Hey! Santa, you flirt! Wait. Take back your chocolate.' I returned it to him. 'Take this also,' and I gave him a few pieces of bubble gum, the ones I used to pop after a quick smoke.

'Attitude!' he bellowed. 'God bless you!'

Towards evening, I could hear the loud music outside my block. We went out to see what was going on. A DJ stood in one corner, playing some rock music, disco lights lit up the surroundings, props were flying all over and it looked as if the whole company was dancing on the floor. Wow! I would say that that was the best thing I had ever seen in my company. That was one good thing about having so many religions represented in one place; there were so many occasions to celebrate. Ali, Subho, Richa and I quickly joined the others, grooving to the dance numbers, while Pritam and Moody stood aloof, looking at each other blankly. I could understand Moody, dancing with rowdy boys to the tunes of desi item numbers would mean she was damaging her family's dignity, but what was Pritam's problem? I guessed the reason. There were invisible sparks flying between him and Moody, but he would never say anything to her. Crazy nerds, both of them! We didn't bother persuading them to join us.

'Hey gal! What are you doing here? Let's join the others and dance.' Of course that wasn't Pritam. Mr Sam made an entry. And no way was Moody going to refuse his offer. Reluctantly, she moved up to the dance floor with Samir holding her hand. Pritam watched Samir in fury, looking like a hungry lion ready to pounce on his prey. A love triangle was taking shape.

But then, it wasn't just Pritam burning that night; Ananya was there too, with her group and with that Gajendra. I still couldn't tolerate the sight of him. After that night when she had introduced me to her ugly sweetheart, I had distanced myself from her. I would visit the gym in the mornings and used my car to commute to work. Whenever she called me out for an afternoon walk, I would excuse myself citing project work. Of late, she had understood and had stopped bothering me. I wondered whether she had noticed my presence there at the Christmas party, but I seriously wished that we wouldn't come face to face. After a while, I grew tired and moved away to light a smoke.

'Cigarette smoking is injurious to health.'

I turned around, Ananya was standing in front of me.

'I know. The statutory warning!' I said.

'I mean it.'

'What?'

'Nothing.'

'Hmm.'

She stood beside silently. Her eyes were compelling me to throw away my cigarette but I didn't want to surrender. And to make it worse, I took a long puff just to show off. I burst into a violent cough when the smoke choked my windpipe. I just couldn't stop coughing.

'I told you it's not good.'

'So, why do you care?'

'Huh! You're angry with me? May I know the reason?'

'Nah! Why would I be angry?'

'Then why are you ignoring me so much?'

'Nothing like that. Just stuck with some work.'

'Whatever. You're just impossible,' she said in disgust.

She walked off.

'Anu! What are you doing here?' That bloody loser Gajendra had followed her.

'Nothing. Let's go. Some people are not worth it,' she said walking away, looking at me, and Gajendra's presence just made it worse.

I chased her down and pulled her by hand. 'Hey! What do you mean by that?' I insisted.

'Gauti, just leave me. Let me go,' she reacted.

'What's happening?' Gajendra followed us. 'What's wrong Ananya?'

'Just fuck off, loser,' I barked at him.

Things between us heated up.

'Ananya! Is he troubling you?'

'Gajendra! Stop! Gauti, leave me.'

'No. Ask him to go. It's between you and me.'

'Gauti! Please let me go. It's hurting,' she cried.

'Let her go,' he demanded and pushed me hard. I lost my balance and fell down.

By that time, Samir had reached the spot. He gave me a hand and pulled me to my feet. He grabbed my arms so that I couldn't attack Gajendra.

'Take her away from here,' Samir said in anger, looking at me. Ananya walked away with that jerk.

'What's this, Gautam?'

'I'll bash that bastard.'

'For what?'

'For…' I paused to look at him. I had no answer.

'Yeah! Dude…for what? Just think what you would have done if someone was stalking Mudrika.'

'I'm not stalking, Ananya. You don't know all that has happened between us,' I said.

'I know it all. Ali told me everything and don't you see that she is playing with you.'

'I don't understand all this.'

'She has a boyfriend and you know that?'

I nodded.

'You still say that you don't understand?'

'But…'

'There should be no BUT in a relationship.'

'So what should I do now?'

'It's your life, you decide. But right now, we are leaving for Goa,' and he beamed.

'Yeah! We are going,' I smiled and we hugged.

When we returned to the dance floor, Moody was already gone. I had missed a chance; I bet she had not danced before in her life. Pritam was relaxed now. Subho was tired. Ali was smoking and Richa was still rocking the dance floor. A few guys had circled her and she was doing her break dance in the centre. A couple of guys tried a few steps just to draw her attention but we knew that would be of no use. We partied for some more time. Ananya had called a few times by then. I had cut her call and Subho had switched off my phone and put it in my pocket.

'I will get the car, you guys bring your stuff to the gate.' I left to fetch my car from the parking lot. I was back in a minute but my friends were yet to come. I took my phone out to call them. They said that they would be there in a moment. As I hung up, I saw a message from Ananya flashing in my inbox. I read it.

'F9 if u don wan 2 talk. I won bother u nymore. M sry 4 watevr hapend dere.'

I should absolutely not call her, a wise voice in my head told me. I threw the phone onto the dashboard. It beeped again.

☹ *at least rply.'*

Those bloody smileys always worked. I cursed their creator before dialling her number.

'Hello!' she picked up at the first ring itself.

'Hi' I said coldly.

'Where are you?'

'I'm in the office campus only, waiting for my friends to come. We are going to Goa tonight for Christmas.'

'Wow! That's awesome, happy journey then.'

'Thanks!'

'How long will you stay there?' she inquired.

'Some four to five days maybe.'

'Then I'll miss you a lot. I want to see you once before you go.'

'Hmm,' I was determined not to get carried away this time. 'I guess that's impossible, I'll leave as soon as my friends come along.'

'But as far as I know, you will have to pass through Panvel only.'

'So?'

'I will wait for you at the station.'

'No. We are not going by train. We have our own car,' I declined straightaway. 'I need to hang up now, my friends are here,' and I cut the call. My friends had arrived and I didn't want another lecture on the issue.

'Let's go to Goa on a holiday!' I exclaimed with energy.

'Amen!' They all cheered in unison.

I exited the campus and drove towards the Goa highway. Metallica played on my music system at a deafening pitch as my friends banged their heads like the hippies; Subho had grown his hair for this very occasion. But somewhere deep down, I kept myself away from the fun because I was driving. But then was I able to concentrate on the road? My mind was still pondering her last line…*I will be waiting for you at the station.* The hoarding on the highway ahead signalled a left turn to Panvel station and a straight route to Goa. *I'm not going to meet her,* I said to myself and accelerated hard, but nearing the left turn, my hand automatically turned the wheel and I could not stop. I was driving at a high speed yet I retained enough control to steer the car well with a sharp turn. Subho, who was sitting next to me, hit his head on the window pane and Ali, who was sitting behind me, tumbled over to Samir sitting at the other end. No casualties though!

'Fuck man! What are you doing?' Subho was terrified.

'Nothing dude! I just want some cigars which won't be available anywhere till we reach Goa,' I said.

'You're mad,' Ali muttered, as he straightened up.

I stopped my car at a good distance from the station so that my friends wouldn't doubt anything. While I was walking towards the station, I thought about it. It was already half an hour past the time that Ananya had told me she would meet me. This was the real test; if I didn't find her there, I would simply close the chapter, I decided. But what if she was there? Was I ready to move on from Riya? For the time being, I knew that I was not worth those thirty minutes that Ananya may have waited.

'Gauti!' Ananya was there.

Though I seriously wanted to put an end to this, I was happy to see her.

'Hi!' I greeted.

'I'm sorry for whatever happened today.'

My smile vanished. 'It's OK,' I said but I still wanted to kill that bastard.

'Happy journey for your trip and enjoy your trip fully.'

'Thank you very much for that. I need to go now. My friends must be waiting for me.'

'Yeah! Sure. Bye,' and she walked away.

I waited below the overbridge as usual for her to wave at me but I could not find her. I didn't notice her in the crowd either. I mean, she had wanted to see me so desperately, yet she showed such attitude. I walked back to my car. I waved out to my friends who were so eagerly waiting for the hundred bucks' worth of smoke. Of course, Subho and Pritam were going to touch a cigar for the first time.

'Gauti! Wait,' Ananya was back and before I could react, she came jogging towards me and gave me a bearhug.

I don't know about my friends but I guess their jaws must have dropped in shock.

'I'll miss you a lot,' she said in my ears.

'Hmm,' I nodded. 'I'll miss you too.'

✍

Nobody asked for the cigar nor did anybody ask about the little romance they had witnessed outside the station. Crazy Metallica droned on for the next four hundred kilometres. They had promised me they wouldn't but one by one, they all dozed off. I was tired too, I had been driving for long, but I didn't want to stop. I wanted to reach Goa as soon as possible and celebrate. But celebrate what?

Hotel Blue Bay at Miramar beach was the destination; it was 6.00 a.m. when we reached. I kicked Subho to wake him up after I had parked the car and then walked to the reception. They all followed me sluggishly with the bags. Samir had already done the booking online for two deluxe rooms. But when I reached the rooms, I could only see one big bed. I flopped down on the bed right away and lay dead to the world.

When I woke up, it was almost noon. All of them were in my room, either in shorts or towels, and were arguing about the schedule for the day. I ignored them and looked around; deluxe facilities gave us a big room, a grand cozy bed, an air conditioner, an LCD TV, a modest sofa and a little refrigerator in the corner. I got out of the bed and opened the fridge. Samir had kept his promise. It was already full. Other than that, what I liked most about that room was the balcony that opened out to a calm and beautiful beach. I put a chair outside and toasted my first drink in Goa.

An hour later, we went out for lunch and then, we were to roam around to explore the place. I checked my phone; there were a few missed calls and messages from Ananya. I read the messages; they all ended with either 'Miss you' or 'Call me back'. I threw my car keys to Samir and called Ananya.

'Good morning!'

'Morning? Baby, it's already two,' she giggled. 'Baby?' Where was this girl leading me? I didn't respond to that.

'Gauti, you must really be having fun there. I wish I was there too.'

'Anu! It's an all boys trip.'

'Hmmm. What will you bring for me from there?'

'What do you want?'

'Feni!' she shouted excitedly.

'You drink? I didn't know that.'

'I am thinking about starting.'

'Starting with Feni? That's pathetic!' I teased.

'Hey! That's my patent line.'

'Whatever.'

'Anyway, if you could really bring something, bring me Jesus' blessings.'

One call to Ananya and time would just fly. I mean, when I had called her, we were still in the hotel and when the car stopped, I realized we had reached Calangute. Was I really on a holiday? We didn't stop talking even then, so I walked with my one hand resting on Pritam walking ahead of me, so that I wouldn't lose them.

We were on the beach when I finally hung up. It was time for some adventure and we explored every option available. The jet-ski ride, the banana ride, the Dolphin safari, parasailing, snorkelling, kayaking, waterskiing and something else that I couldn't recall later, although it was actually the best one. Two of us were made to sit on a water tube and were dragged outrageously far out into the sea, towed by a motor boat. We had to do nothing but hold on. I was with Subho and when I looked at him, I thought his heart was almost in his mouth. He had closed his eyes and gripped the tube so tight, his face was pale and his body was numb. With a push, the ride began and along with it, a loud cry from Subho also began, which only ended when the motor boat stopped. Occasionally, I would scare him by shaking him by the hand and he would get the scare of his life and shiver even more.

If the days were given to those scary rides, the nights were for rocking the local discos and pubs. We had already decided that once in Goa, we would only drink neat. No water, no soda. I don't remember any of us drinking anything other than alcohol, not even water, in our entire time in Goa. Even the food was quite wild. We experimented and sampled everything, right from octopus to snail. In one such large-hearted mood, we ordered squid, which everyone relished, but later, when I showed them the creature on Discovery channel, Pritam turned vegetarian for life.

But the best thing I remember about Pritam was the night we spent on the beach. We were so drunk that none of us was in a state to drive back to the hotel. It was cold out there under the night sky which looked like a grand dome covered with little lights. The darker the sky got, the closer and clearer the stars appeared. So many stars—mysterious, eerie, calm, tranquil, but most of all, entrancing. You couldn't help but wonder if there is other life up there, whether you are significant in any way in the universe. It was amazing to sit gazing up at the sky and I understood why the night sky is equated with romance. For miles around, it was silent, with the only sound being the rhythm of waves in the mighty sea. We sat shivering in the cool breeze and even the sand felt like ice. Alcohol was the only way for us to survive. We had stocked up well for the night ahead. We drank beyond our limits that night, until our hands were so unsteady we couldn't even pick up our glasses.

'So this goes for Gautam, who finally managed to get a hug from his love,' Subho announced.

'Dude! I don't love her,' I protested. 'I just want to sleep with her.'

'Is it?' Samir burped. I nodded.

'Bhai! She is so smart…'

'I know she is using me and blah blah…' I interrupted. 'Anything else you guys want to say?'

'We are your friends…'

'So? Can't we talk about something else?'

'Like what?'

'I mean, has anyone ever bothered to think about Pritam?'

'What about him?'

'Does anybody know about his silent romance?' I asked. Pritam gave me a blank look. He was probably angry with me for spilling the beans or maybe it was simply the alcohol effect. Perhaps, I thought, he had always wanted this issue to be discussed so that he could take a stand. Like me, his love story wasn't going anywhere, although he clearly loved Moody from day one.

'Moody?!' Everyone looked in astonishment.

'Yes!' I declared.

Everyone now looked at Pritam. This was one of those situations when he might have seriously wished that dinosaurs still roamed the planet and found him and gobbled him up. He was expecting some motivation, tips, support or at least consolation, but like him, his emotions also were ignored.

'Thinking of him and her, Mr Dumb with Miss Best, there is no doubt in my mind that their children would be the dumbest people on earth,' Ali joked and everyone roared with laughter.

This statement didn't go down well with Pritam and was silent (though being silent was normal for him) and walked some distance away from us, along the water's edge.

'Hey bro!' I went to him. 'What's wrong?'

He remained quiet, watching the beach.

'Listen! Moody is no big deal. You can get a better girl than her,' I said, because I very well knew that Pritam simply couldn't get Moody.

He replied in a stern voice. 'That's the truth. You know nothing about her.'

You see, there are only two types of honest people in this world, small children and drunken guys. So, being one of them, I just went on.

'You also know her obsessive behaviour of always trying to be the best.' He nodded. 'I mean, this craving of hers to be the best is way too childish and irritating. And in that bid, she sometimes feels low that she does not have a boyfriend and so she stalks almost all the good guys around. Right now she is into Samir, you know that. They have been quite close these days. I mean, I even saw Samir talking to her yesterday, late in the night. Though Samir is ok! But the reason behind her pursuing him is not OK. She is kinda desperate about it. Who knows if tomorrow someone else seems even better, Moody will surely drift again, and why do you think we call her Moody. And trust me buddy, I know how it feels when your heart is broken,' I concluded.

He didn't reply. Anyway I did not expect him to say anything. He was like that. Calm and silent or you could say foolish and dumb. He was still looking at the sea. I could sense the defeat in him, tears filled his eyes and in another moment, a stream came flowing down. Love sucks, I thought.

It was hard seeing him like that. I wondered whether I should console him or let him cry or tease him again. But my phone chose that moment to ring. *Ananya calling.* So there I was, giving him a tedious lecture about moving on from loving a girl and now, I was going to leave him alone when he most needed me, for another girl.

'Hey!' she said cheerfully.

'Hi Anu! What's up?'

'Nothing much, the ceiling and the bloody old fan.'

'What?'

'You asked na, what's up?' She giggled.

'That was Pathetic!'

'Hey! That's my patent word. Anyway, what about you?'

'I'm fine.'

'Stupid, I'm asking what's up?'

'Oh! It's a dark and silent night sky with enchanting little stars peering at us from afar.'

'You're in the balcony?'

'Nah! Can't you hear the waves behind me?'

'Hey! You're on the beach!'

'Hmmm.'

'Wow! At this time?' She was excited. It was two at night.

'So?'

'You on that beach, me here, at this time, sounds so romantic!' She chuckled. 'I want to hear the waves.'

'OK!' I went closer to the water, with the waves lapping my feet. It sent a chill down my body. Hate you Ananya!

'I can't hear it!' she complained. 'Go closer.'

'Are you mad?'

'Closer!' she demanded.

I extended my hand closer. One big wave and my iPhone would be gone, but then, guys actually can't do anything about such stupid tantrums.

'Wow! This sound is so mesmerizing! Thank you Gautam!' she said. 'I wish I were there with you right now. We would've held hands and walked on the beach...'

I could only grunt in reply. I mean what was she up to? She didn't talk or meet for a week, then insulted me. Two hours later, she was waiting for me at the station, and then that hug. She messaged me all the time that she was missing me and now we were chatting so late in night. Durjoy Dutta says if you exchange more than twenty-five messages a day or talk at least two hours on the phone everyday, then you're in love. So was one of us in love? Me or she?

Office Shocks

I sat in office, uploading our photos of the Goa trip on Facebook. There was only one word to describe those photos—marvellous. You see, you won't find a single IT guy who's not been to Goa with his office colleagues and then posted an album called Go Goa on Facebook. A lot of things changed between us after that trip. We now understood and respected each other better and loved each other even more than before. I never thought Pritam could be such a softie, Samir indeed had all the qualities we were jealous of, it was not safe to be with Ali alone and Subho was actually a nice guy but I still doubted his engineering degree, he knew nothing! On our return journey, our car had broken down due to overheating and there was no water around. Looking for water on that deserted road after midnight was an adventure in itself. I would cherish these memories all my life.

'Hey! Did you see it?' Subho came running to my desk.

'What?'

'Samir just updated his status on Facebook to "In a relationship",' he said excitedly.

So what was I supposed to do? Jump onto my desk, hug Samir or cry for Moody? I gave Subho a blank look.

'Fuck man! Don't you wanna know with whom?'

I shook my head, 'Do I care?'

'Then you must,' he said. He had a sly smile that resembled Muthu's smile and I hated it. I went back to my screen.

'Dude, see if Samir has updated it then Moody has definitely seen it. I mean, she stalks his profile all day, so she should be like crying or yelling, instead she has been smiling all day.'

'So what does that tell you?' I was baffled, Subho was so irritating.

'She might be the girl!'

'Are you mad?' I snapped. 'Boss! He is Samir, perfect material for a Raymond ad and she is Miss Drama Queen, *dehati* turned modern. It's not possible.'

'You're not getting my point,' Subho argued.

'Whatever, I'll just ask Samir during lunch. Now piss off.'

So it was official now. Subho was right, Moody and Samir were now a couple. But how did it happen? I asked Richa about it. She told me that Moody had asked him on Facebook whether he had a girlfriend and Samir had replied that he was single. Moody then told him that it was hard to believe that a guy like Samir was single, to which Samir answered that if she was so concerned, why didn't she become his girlfriend. Moody sent a smiley in response followed by a 'yes' in all CAPS. Listening to this story, all of us looked at each other blankly. It was like Samir setting out on his bike alone and Moody asking him to give her a lift instead of going solo. It was simply ridiculous.

'Desperate wannabe!' we all shouted in unison.

I realized that Pritam was not in the office. Just as Subho had come to me, he must have told Pritam too. Poor Pritam's heart must have broken. We decided to leave him alone for some time. Yet, in a way, I was happy for him; Moody didn't deserve him. She was too blind to see his true love. But then in today's world, true love was just not enough. Samir threw a small treat for the group and we joined the new couple. After all, it was meant for Moody and she was a dear friend. And we felt that was the end of all fun, so we celebrated it.

∽

Things changed drastically after that day. Samir became a regular in our group. He was with us everywhere—at lunch, on outings, while shopping and even during gossip sessions. Even when he didn't want to be with us, Moody would drag him along. She wanted him to be a part of the group but that would hurt Pritam, which was unacceptable to the rest of us. He overworked, skipped lunch and avoided our company. Day by day, Samir's dominance in the group left us suffocating but all of us remained silent for Moody's sake.

'Hey! What's for lunch today?' Subho asked. 'Didn't you order rice?'

'Actually, Samir placed the order,' Richa said.

'OK! Samir, didn't you order rice?'

He completely ignored Subho, he was busy cuddling Moody at the corner of the table.

'Samir!' Richa's voice rose a pitch and both of them immediately turned to look. Nobody messed with her. 'Subho is asking something.'

'Yes! I didn't. Rice is unhealthy. C'mon dude! Get out of this stupid Bong habit,' he said curtly.

Subho didn't reply but he was visibly hurt. Moody was unfazed as if nothing was wrong in Samir's words. That was enough for me, I couldn't see my friends hurt like that. I walked to the counter and picked up a rice plate.

'What are you trying to prove?' Moody asked me since I had clearly challenged her darling's authority.

'Nothing. I just want to eat what I want and not what someone else decides.'

'Gauti, I very well understand what you mean by that. Mind it. I won't tolerate it next time,' an argument was brewing.

'C'mon, honey! Chill. They are your friends.'

After the thunder comes the storm.

'Samir! You dare not poke your fucking head into this. It's between the group,' Richa blasted him. That stunned Samir and set him back, but his saviour took the lead.

'What's this, Richa? How can you talk like that to Samir?'

'And didn't you see how he talked to Subho?'

'He just said it sarcastically, he didn't mean it.'

'But I mean what I said, every bit of it. It's high time now. He might be your boyfriend but that doesn't mean that he can insult us and boss our lives.'

'Shut up, Richa! You people are so narrow-minded and mean.

You just can't see me happy.'

The argument was now growing into a big fight and I was pretty confident that one more such line from Moody and we would see Samir dead on the floor. You never knew with Richa's violent streak. However, I desperately wanted to witness something like that. I really wished to see Samir in a pool of blood and Moody crying beside him, but Subho intervened.

'That's enough people! Stop it. Let's not create a scene here. Sit down.'

'No. I won't sit here. This table is too fucking small for all of us. Who the hell selected this one?' Richa demanded but nobody answered. We already knew it, we looked at Moody and Samir.

'What? Samir said that the AC temperature is just fine here,' Moody justified.

'Gosh! Moody, fuck off.'

We left them and shifted to another table. Subho had his rice, Richa had her frustration vented and Ali finally pulled out his earphones, freaked out by the scene. We had a silent lunch, nobody discussed anything, and yet there was a common conclusion that Moody was out from our group. Later on in the evening, we forced Pritam to stop working, drove to my flat, drank Old Monk, slept and forgot everything.

∽

Pritam was back with us. We thought that things would slowly fall in place again but that didn't seem likely anytime soon. Maybe you couldn't get away easily after insulting a senior's girlfriend who happened to be from the same village as your manager, the one who thinks you're good for nothing. Office politics is bad, especially when you have stuck your ass in it. We were shifted to the database and were given two weeks to clean up data that had been accumulated over a period of ten years. No human being could have done that. Forget about completing it, taking up the task itself should have given us an entry into the Guinness Book of World Records. We complained with teary eyes but we were made to remember those nine promises of IT from chapter eight, remember? (Not everything in this book is fiction, you see.)

'Richa, can you get me some coffee?' I requested.

'No man! I'm too tired to walk till the pantry,' she refused. It was already nearing dawn but we hadn't managed to finish the task.

'What's your status?'

'Another one and half hour to two hours and I'll meet my target for the day,' she said.

'What about you three?'

Listening to the others, I realized I was way behind target. You really can't work with Akon blasting in your ears. Moreover, I was tired. It was hard for me to keep my eyelids from falling, forget about continuing the work. Three to four hours of sleep and one lunch per day was just not enough to support a one hundred and sixty pound frame, that too after a double shift of labour and two hours of driving. I had forgotten when I last used my dining table at home. Mornings were never normal, it was always a mad rush where I had hardly fifteen minutes to get ready, and I was determined not to take a bath until this project was closed.

'Hey! I'm leaving. I'll come early tomorrow. I desperately need sleep.' I bid my friends goodbye and drove back home at full speed. The last thing I remember from that night was struggling to get my keys to open the locked door of home sweet home.

∽

It was seven in the morning when I reached office the next day. For people like us, it feels like the middle of the night. Anyway, I still had three hours to complete the target. I motivated myself somehow, it felt like I was appearing for some board exam and trust me, I had never worked so hard before for anything. Sometime, I seriously considered paying the bond amount and switching to another company but then my friends couldn't do that, so I continued wagging my tail for our pig.

The campus was almost empty, with only a few BPO guys loitering about and the security personnel at work. My department would definitely be empty; those losers never turned up before 10.30. To avoid distraction, I hadn't charged my iPod. So that in three hours, with no disturbance, I would surely get the work done.

For about half an hour, everything was going well, but then I began feeling restless. I tried to concentrate on the screen but something was bothering me. It was as if I could feel somebody's presence around me. And that thought freaked me out. I had heard stories of the campus having been developed where once there had been a graveyard, and people staying back alone in the building had complained of many strange things happening.

It's just an illusion. Ghosts are like engineers, inactive in the mornings, I comforted myself. Yet that strange feeling continued to haunt my mind. I took a break to light a cigarette. On my way out, I noticed that the light in the server room was on. Pritam must have mistakenly left it on, I wondered. Or it was just a trap set up by the so-called 'ghosts'. I ignored it. I stood outside for a while and finished my cigarette. Walking back to my desk, my attention turned once more to the light in the server room. This time, I decided I had had enough; I couldn't work like that with my mind full of those stupid doubts. I was going in there and switching off that little light.

I swiped my card and the door opened. I moved towards the switchboard when I sensed a familiar scent in the room. Next, I saw a bag lying on a chair and I knew very well to whom it belonged. I was now all the more curious and wanted to find out what was going on. I tiptoed silently to the darker side of the room where unused and malfunctioning equipment were dumped. And what did I see there?

I ran out of the room and out of my department as fast as I could. Once out of the building, I stood panting, taking deep breaths. I wished I had not gone in there, it would have been better if I had seen a ghost and not what I did see. It couldn't be true, I said to myself, but I had witnessed it with my own eyes—Moody and Samir, stark naked, making out!

It gave me such a shock, I sat under a tree until I returned to my senses. I was not sure if they had noticed me. What was I supposed to do now? I called Richa. What would I say to her, that I had caught them in the act? Gosh! How could Moody be such a moron? What if somebody else had caught them? What would her parents think about this? Ultimately, I didn't tell Richa anything. I would never tell anyone about this incident.

Now, the next big question was how would I face them? I thought about waiting somewhere outside till my friends came to the office. I looked at my watch, it was 7.45 a.m. Two hours more to go. I couldn't wait that long. Then I wondered why I was freaking out. I mean, I wasn't the one doing anything wrong. I wasn't caught in the act. It was they who should be afraid. Perhaps, I could even blackmail Samir and put ourselves out of our work misery, but what about Moody? I still cared for her. *Stupid girl!*

Slowly, I walked backed to my department. Moody was sitting at her desk with a blank expression, Samir was nowhere to be seen. I didn't say anything and went straight to my desk. Moody remained that way for some time before bursting into tears. I looked around, Samir was still missing but I decided it was better to leave her alone.

'Gauti, I know what you must be thinking right now,' she sobbed. I didn't respond.

'I'm a slut.'

'Shut up! Moody. Are you out of your mind?'

'We love each other.'

'Well…what I saw wasn't love, we call it lust.'

'What could I do? I don't want to lose him. I will do anything for him. Because it's just he who cares for me now, you people have deserted me completely. I hate you all.'

'You know why we left you. We don't like him.'

'So, it's a choice between you guys and Samir?' she paused. 'I choose him over you all because I love him.'

'Your wish. Your life. But next time, be careful.'

That was it, we didn't talk again about it and neither did she cry again. She went out after that and only returned around 10.30

with Samir. She seemed normal as if nothing had happened, but her words rang in my ears, hurting me so much. Was it our fault? We left her alone and it was easy for Samir to tame her but neither was she a kid nor would we have snubbed her if she had come to us. I didn't know what was right and what was wrong. Moreover, I couldn't even convince my heart in this matter. I decided to keep it a secret.

∞

A few days later, things started to change. The pressure on us slackened. What had been hyped as such an important project was closed without any notice and we could finally breathe easy. Everyone was happy and moved on but only I knew what a big price we had paid for it. After that incident, I had hacked Moody's company profile and checked her timings. I realized that what I had seen was just one of many such morning sessions. If rumours were to be believed, she had started going on holidays with Samir, lying at home that she was on business tours. In a way, we were responsible for it all, we had ruined that simple-minded little girl. I missed the old Moody so much.

One afternoon, Ananya and I were out for a walk when she suddenly brought up the subject.

'Hey! What's up with Moody? I haven't seen her with you all for quite some time.'

I just nodded.

'The other day, I saw her with a guy in the mall.'

'He must be Samir, her beau.'

'Wow! That's awesome, they looked great together. She was so happy.'

That hurt. I knew that happiness of that sort didn't last long. Over the past few days, I had done quite a bit of detailed research on him and the results weren't pleasing. Moody was hardly the first girl in his life, he was a womanizer. I found out about many of his popular romantic stints from his previous office and I was actually worried about Moody. The worst thing I learned was that he was planning to shift to the US and Moody was still unaware. I did want to tell

Moody everything because I was afraid that it would only backfire on me; Moody was so much into him.

I was lost in a stream of thoughts and Ananya had to shake me to catch my attention.

'What's wrong, Gauti?'

I smiled and said, 'It's all fine.'

But I had so much on my mind that I had been feeling suffocated lately and knew I needed to clear my head. I just had to get that monkey off my back, so I told her everything.

'Oh my God! The girl is going this wild? She needs your help, you should talk to her,' she was overreacting.

'I don't feel the situation is that tense, it's not a big deal these days. Everybody does it.' I hadn't meant to hint at Ananya but she took it the other way.

'What do you mean by that statement of yours, Mr Gautam Deshmukh?' she asked angrily.

I shook my head, 'Nothing personal.'

'Girls are not like that. You guys run behind us for that.' Now the conversation was shaping up very badly.

So I hit back, 'Is it? Don't tell me you never did it. I mean, four years is quite long.'

'Yes! We haven't done anything yet and that's what I like about him. He is not after me for sex, he genuinely loves me.'

'Hah! You're a jackpot for him and he fears losing you. So he doesn't have the guts to do it.'

'I am afraid you're totally wrong. Actually, we've never even got such a chance. The day we get such a chance, I mean, like a night out together, then probably…'

'That's my point,' I cut in.

She gave me a look of hatred. 'You're such a disgusting fellow. Go to hell.' And she ran away.

I wasn't really panicking though that had become a regular pattern with us by then. A maximum of two days would pass and then she would herself call me. Anyway, she had told me something important.

I had to talk to Moody about Samir.

∞

Back in the office, I didn't talk about it to anyone. I was waiting for an opportunity to talk to her privately but it was quite difficult now, since we were not friends anymore and even the slightest move on my part would have attracted attention. So I had to be very cautious. I followed her when she headed to the restroom and waited for her outside. She came out after a full half hour; I always wonder what girls do so much inside.

'Moody! I need to talk.' I cornered her.

'What?'

'About Samir.'

'What?' This time there was an intensity in her voice.

'He is not a nice guy.'

'What?' Her voice got louder. Another 'What?' and I was to go straight to my desk. 'Do you know that he is going to the US?'

She shook her head. 'What?' Now her voice had dropped to a low pitch and she looked genuinely surprised.

'Go and ask him about it.'

She gave me an uncertain look and walked off. I heaved a sigh of relief. Finally, I felt that I was heading the right way. Things would be alright again.

The very next day, the first thing I did after coming to office was to ping her.

'Asked?'

'Yes, meet me outside in sometime.'

☺'

She didn't reply.

I stepped out of the office, signalling her to follow. I waited for her in the smoking zone. At that early hour, it was empty. Moody came down shortly. Her expression was not pleasing, she was fuming but I ignored it, thinking that I was finally going to get my old dear friend back.

'What did he say?'

'A lot.'

'Really?'

'He told me what you told him in Goa.' She sobbed. Samir had taken up the fight well, I could see. 'What did he say?'

'That I'm *despo* and *chep*, I run behind every guy and Pritam was lucky that I was not with him.'

Now, every bit of it was true yet I reckoned that I had got myself into big trouble. I couldn't believe that the bastard had used this against me. I was just helping Pritam. I knew I would never be able to explain that to her. I was dead.

'See Moody, I was drunk that night,' I defended.

'So what? You will talk nonsense about me?' She was now howling. I prayed that no one would see us then. People would think I was trying to rape her.

'Listen Moody, you're getting it all wrong. That asshole is misleading...'

A tight slap was planted on my right cheek before I could complete my sentence.

'You dog! Don't you dare say anything about him! I now know everything about you guys. You people do nothing other than smoking, drinking and bitching about others.'

'Moody...'

My left cheek came next. Moody was not in the mood to stop, she was on a mission that day. Destroy Gautam!

'And about America, he didn't tell me because he wanted to give me a surprise. We are moving soon.'

Down the Road

I couldn't find my feet. I felt so weak within that I collapsed on the floor. She had slapped my face but I could feel the pain somewhere deep inside in my heart. I was shaking with the humiliation of what had just happened. I had only wanted to help, I cared for her. And this was what I had got in return—a sense of utter disgrace that made me feel awful about myself. What if anybody had seen us? What would people think of me? It's always the guy who is at fault. Moreover, how would I face myself in the mirror? A moment later, I saw my friends running towards me. So the news was out on the floor already. I couldn't possibly work there anymore. It would all be over in a moment.

'Gauti! Gauti!' Ali shook me.

'Say something!' Subho screamed. I was still on the floor, numb. 'Are you alright?'

I was crying. Pritam gave me a hug while the others waited for me to feel better.

'How can you cry like that? You're a man,' Richa said.

I couldn't even see her clearly, my eyes were brimming over with tears. I felt a tightness in my chest, I still didn't have the strength to stand up. A part of me had died. Murdered, perhaps.

'I just couldn't believe it when she called me into the washroom and told me about this,' Richa recalled.

'She is so insensitive and mean. See, what she did to him,' Ali said.

'She is a bitch. I wondered what stopped me from dunking her head in the toilet but I will not spare her this time,' Richa swore.

'No Richa! You're doing nothing,' Subho piped in.

'Why Subho? Why?' she bawled.

'We cannot let this episode get out. That will only tamper Gauti's image and she will get a little warning, max to max.'

'You mean we should let that fucking slut merrily get away with her pimp.'

'I don't know but my intuition says we should stay quiet for now. We will see her once the right time comes. As of now, think about Gauti! We will talk about this later,' Subho suggested.

'But…' Richa protested.

'See, whatever she did was wrong. But we just can't let this news get out because that will only hamper his name further. Anyway, girls are never at fault and Samir is with her.'

It took me a few days to recover from the incident but it had left a mark on me for life, neither could I forget it nor was I to forgive. But there wasn't much that we could have done. The events of that day had an impact on both sides. A cold war had begun between the weak and the strong. Yes! We were the weaker ones. Samir, Moody, Muthu and a few seniors from their side were in one league and we were stuck in a shit-hole. But we were far more determined to hang in there, and this time round, the bond was the trump card. We couldn't be sacked for at least one year without a valid reason. However, with passing time, I started to feel the heat. I felt bad for my friends, the onus was actually on me but my friends had to suffer it too. Quitting the job and moving to another place would be a sign of cowardice. I wanted to fight back but I didn't want to be the reason for my friends' miseries. I was the source of the problem, it was better that I stayed aloof.

It was a slow process but eventually, I got out of it. The office was not a place to hang out anymore, we only worked there. Those chirpy chats and blabbering were extinct. The casualness in our body language was gone. There was a new code of discipline we followed. We wore formals to office. Lunch was the only time when we met each other but we ordered our food separately. We broke up. The Super-Six team was dead and buried.

Pritam had applied to the army and was selected for the SSB. Subho got busy writing his novel. Richa's parents were keen on getting her married by the end of the year, so most her time was spent on matrimonial sites while Ali, they say, got a boyfriend. Mine was the worst case. I had nothing to do and my loneliness started to kill me. Ananya was the only option I had and I completely surrendered to her. It was actually during this time that I started to think about her more seriously. Sachin's marketing job had kept Ananya away from him for a while, so I would have the opportunity to ease myself back into her life, I thought. But it turned out the other way.

We travelled together, went out for dinners, roamed around in the malls, shopped a lot and also went to Essel World. Life with her was crazy. I mean, who would ask you out on a trip to Essel World for a romantic date? Ananya was *that* unpredictable. Then one day, she wanted to smoke but couldn't go beyond a puff, she coughed badly till her face turned red. I teased her for being so coy and to prove herself, she actually smoked five cigarettes that evening. She even wanted to booze but I had always ignored her request, thinking of the side-effects. With her, happiness came into my life once again, after our group had split up. Our relationship was growing gradually, our feelings for each other started to deepen. She occasionally held my hand and we hugged each other at every instance. The physical barrier between us was overcome but I wondered when we would cross the line. Actually, I feared losing her. I didn't know what she felt for me. Maybe I wasn't sure of my own mind, did I love her yet or did I only want to sleep with her.

∽

'Gosh! They made you go naked,' Ali exclaimed. 'Do they want soldiers or porn stars?'

Pritam had returned from his SSB interview, he was rejected for his crooked index finger. It was a big disappointment since he had always dreamt of being an army man. So we arranged a small get-together at my place to cheer him up.

'It's for the medical test stupid, just to check that you don't have any abnormalities in your body,' Subho explained.

'Hmm,' Ali grunted. I'm positive he was desperately thinking of appearing for the army exam too, not for a job or anything, just for the medical test.

'Hey guys! I'm bored. Do you have any movies?' Richa put down her glass. Four large RC and one quarter bottle of White Mischief with Limca but I was sure she was not done yet.

'Just go into the bedroom, you will find my laptop somewhere,' I pointed her the way towards the room.

'OK,' she rose and went to get the laptop.

'Gauti,' she shouted from the room, 'Do you have a mouse? I am not comfortable with the touch pad.'

'It's OK! Bring it here, I've got something better for you,' I answered.

She brought out the laptop and gave it to me. I switched on the power button and waited for it to boot.

'Gauti, I told you I need a mouse.'

'There is no need for it in my laptop, I've got Sunayana in my laptop.'

'Who is she? Pornstar? Indian?' Subho's eyes were filled with joy. He had this fondness for Indian stuff.

'No dude! It's my final year project.'

'What?' Everyone took a closer look at my laptop.

'Well, this is an interface which tracks eye movements and can be used to direct the pointer. So, no need of a mouse or a touchpad, Richa,' I explained.

'This is really good,' Richa said as she tried it while the others looked on curiously.

'This is not just good. This is brilliant, even Steve Jobs doesn't have it,' I said it with a touch of pride. I admired and loved my baby.

'Wow! Gauti! You're so talented. Why the hell are you wasting yourself here?'

'Because I don't want to leave you guys,' I said, smiling sarcastically.

'That's too senti! Fuck off, Gauti,' Richa retorted while we all had a hearty laugh.

We watched *Batman Begins*, Subho's favourite. Whenever we watched a movie on a laptop and Subho was around, it had to be this one or its sequel. I wondered how many more times he would watch them, he knew all the dialogues by heart.

'Eureka! I've got an idea for Gautam,' Subho screamed.

'Don't tell me you want me to become a Batman.'

'Of course not! But I got something from the movie.'

'What?'

'Gautam can start his own business of developing applications. Anyway, he has nothing to do after office.'

'Sounds good but I won't do it alone, I need some help.'

'We are with you, bro,' Ali announced his support.

'Yes! Then we can have our own company.'

'Company? Applications? And sell what and to whom?'

'IT solutions dude, a little consultancy type of thing.'

'And where do we get our clients from?' inquired Richa.

'We can bag quite a few deals from our company itself. See, most of the development tasks of our company are outsourced, we can get them,' Subho suggested.

'And how will you do this? I mean, do you think Mr Bose will pay his own employees for these applications.'

'Boss! That's where lies the intellectual difference between us and them.'

'What do you mean?'

'See, its age of e-commerce, clients need not see their vendors. We are just a company with no face. We will operate as freelance developers.'

'Again the question arises, why would Mr Bose be interested in us. He might have bigger names around him.'

'That could actually hamper our chances but we can at least try. You see, I overheard Mr Bose's conversation on the phone the other day. Samir's project is going nowhere. They plan to outsource it and if that happens, he will soon be kicked out of the office.'

'Is it?' Now I was curious.

Subho nodded.

'Then leave it to me, I'll handle the publicity.'

∽

Life is easy when you have a rich and influential dad. I called him the very next day and told him about our venture idea. He was very amused to know our plans and extended his full support. He told me that he would register our company in Pune and provide me with documents and certificates which would prove that we had been a helping hand behind his wi-fi venture in the city and that would truly boost our popularity.

'How about Batman IT Solutions?' Subho suggested the name for the company. 'I mean, we are like him. We work in the night and are all set to kick that Joker, Samir, off the planet.'

'Grow up boy! You're not an American burger-hogging teenager,' I teased him.

'I guess Cherry is fine. Steve Jobs has Apple and ours is just a small venture. It will have great attitude and energy.'

'No. The name should be something different and carry some weight. It should be Indian. I say Vighnam.'

'What does that mean, Richa?' we all growled in chorus.

'I have the best name,' it was Ali's turn. 'Masti IT Solutions.'

'Are you kidding me? Is this a name for an IT Company?' I protested right away.

'Masti IT Solutions is perfect, it's a very catchy name. It will draw attention instantly,' Ali argued.

'Gosh! We are here to decide a brand name for an IT company and not a condom,' I was baffled.

∽

In a week, everything was set. We did the registration, got the required documents and also worked on the publicity. We did our homework perfectly and were ready to start. Subho's years of goodwill came in handy. He was able to divert Mr Bose's attention to our plan. He was a bit apprehensive to trust a newbie like us but comparatively low market rates and Dad's testimonies worked in our favour. We had insisted on no physical meetings, on carrying out every procedure via emails or calls, citing our busy schedule. 'Payment only after delivery' was our policy; that was the only way we could win Mr Bose's trust. And we got our first deal.

A month later, when I checked the post box, we had a letter addressed to us. I opened the envelope. It carried a cheque of one lakh rupees, drawn in favour of Masti IT Solutions.

Mom Says No Girlfriend!

I woke up early with the sound of my cell phone ringing but I cut the call. I wanted to sleep some more. The past few days, our work had stretched quite long into the nights. We had bagged most of the available assignments after our initial success. The secret to our success was the fact that our products hardly ever had bugs in them and were cleared in the first check itself. And why wouldn't it be so? We developed the applications at home during the night and reviewed them in the office in the morning. And the funny thing was that we were paid for both.

I couldn't go back to sleep. I checked my phone, the call had been from Mom. I called her back.

'Hello Mom!'

'Hello beta! How are you?'

'Mom, I'm fine. I was sleeping,' I complained.

'Sorry but I was missing you a lot. Nandita came home last night for the weekend. I wish you were here too. It's been a while since you visited us. Don't you care for us anymore?' Mom and her emotional atyachar.

'Mom! Stop it now. I'll see, maybe tomorrow morning. I want to sleep now…bye.'

'Beta, wait. Listen!' she wasn't finished but I cut the call and dozed off again.

It was Saturday and I slept almost all day. Late in the day, again I was woken up by a call. This time it was Ananya. I picked it up.

'Hey, Gauti!' I wondered why she was so cheerful all the time.

'Hi Anu!' I tried to match up to her level of cheerfulness.

'What's up?'

'Nothing re. I'm still in bed, slept all day.'

'Boy! You're so lazy.'

I grunted and it went on. When I cut the call, I checked the call duration. One hour and forty-five minutes. I recalled that Mom's call had lasted a mere forty-five seconds. Girls are true time devils.

It really had been long since I had been home and now that Didi was there too, I actually looked forward to it. It's not that I didn't like going home but then that lonely drive of three hours from Mumbai to Pune and then another three hours to get back simply sucked. I could talk to her over Skype, I thought. However, I was missing them badly and I was also fed up of Kantabai's dull and tasteless food.

I called all my friends but everyone seemed to refuse, citing their own personal engagements. That left me with only one option— Ananya Singh. So I called her up and asked her to be ready early in the morning. I had a big surprise for her, I told her. I knew how valuable those sleep-till-late-Sundays were but I also knew girls always have a soft corner for surprises. And she had not yet seen my Rampyari!

∽

'Wow! Nice car,' she had a big smile seeing my baby. 'Whose car is this?'

I flashed her a big grin.

'Where are we going?' she asked as she got into the car.

'Well, that's a surprise.'

'Is it?' she smiled and went on to check out the buttons on the dashboard.

'This car really seems great but I think it's too small like the Nano on the inside.'

That gave me a shock and I almost hit the brake. It was an insult to my baby.

'Anu! This is a Volkswagen Beetle convertible. You can buy more than twenty Nanos with this single one.'

Her jaw dropped.

'Gauti! Did you steal this car?' she asked me anxiously.

'Anu! Why don't you enjoy some light music and relax?'

I played some soothing oldies and turned on the AC. We got stuck in traffic because of some construction work which actually kept me occupied, as I used my all experience with the steering wheel to escape the jam. And when I finally got the car out on the expressway, Ananya had already dozed off.

Once on the expressway, there was no looking back. I stayed well over 120km/hr all the way to Pune, even the dangerous Khandala Ghats couldn't deter my spirits. As a child, I had dreamt of becoming an F1 driver but Dad hadn't allowed me to pursue it later.

When Ananya woke up, we were in the outskirts of Pune.

'Where are we?' she asked.

'Pune.'

'What?' she screamed. 'Are you kidding me?'

I pointed to the sign board of a little shop carrying the city name.

'What's this? You're kidnapping me or what?' she asked. I looked at her to see whether she had said that sarcastically. But she had a blank expression on her face.

'C'mon Ananya! I swear, this is my car.'

She made a face.

'I know it's hard to believe but I have a rich dad.'

'You never told about this,' she still could not believe me.

'I did tell you about Deshmukh Finance in our first meeting itself but you just snubbed me.'

She tried to recall but couldn't.

'Why didn't you tell me later?'

'I thought that wasn't necessary. You tell me, do you see any change in me after knowing that I'm rich.'

'I don't know,' she shook her head.

We didn't discuss it further; I got busy evading Pune traffic. She sat silently, looking out of the window. She reminded me of a similar situation I had been in before. Two girls didn't like me for being rich. One of them had already dumped me and I wondered what this one was thinking about. Damn it! Who said girls loved rich guys?

Being rich seemed to be the biggest curse of my life but I couldn't help it. Just like you couldn't choose your religion, race or creed, you couldn't choose being born rich or poor. I was regretting telling Ananya about it; I couldn't afford to lose her. She meant a lot to me. She meant everything to me.

My car reached the gate of our mansion. I honked and the doorman opened it. As I drove in, I looked at her again. She was still silent but her mouth was wide open and her eyes were full of wonder at the beautiful and bright flowers in the garden and the splendid big mansion ahead. I stopped beside the fountain and gestured to her to open the door.

'Gauti, should I tell you something?' she said as she got out of the car.

I nodded.

'You're not rich but super rich,' she was giggling when she said that. I really didn't know whether that statement was a compliment or a taunt. Had I actually impressed her or did she too think that I was a rich spoilt brat, a good-for-nothing.

I gave her a smile and drove off to park the car in the garage. When I came back, she was on an exploring spree in the garden. Mom loved gardening and we had some really great varieties to flaunt. Until that point, I was rather convinced that the fact that I was rich didn't have any negative impact on her. And of course, that led me to my next thought—would she now love me just because I had big money? God! Being rich was such a bane.

∞

'Hey Mom! I'm home, where are you all?' I yelled. That was my standard greeting every time I had returned home from school or college.

Everyone was upstairs. When they heard my voice, they rushed out and watched from the railings. They had a big smile on their face, seeing me after such a long time, but their smiles vanished when they noticed Ananya. I guess she didn't realize that. She had a sheepish little smile on her face. They all came down and we had a big family bear hug. Didi and I had particularly hated that as children but those days were different; now the *jaadu ki jhappi* always worked. Ananya watched us, amazed to see our filmy style of greeting each other. She felt left out.

'Mom! This is Ananya. She is my colleague,' I introduced.

'Hello beta! How do you do?' Mom greeted her warmly.

'I'm fine Aunty. How are you?'

They all exchanged smiles and introductions were made.

It was almost lunch time. Ananya and I freshened up and joined the others at the table. Mom had cooked all my favourite dishes. I missed her food so much. *I love you Mom.*

∽

'Don't tell me Uncle, you actually did that?' Ananya laughed. Dad was telling us old tales from his youth about how Mom and he had got together. We had grown up hearing those stories several times but we never minded hearing them repeatedly. Dad had this knack of entertaining people, especially women. I could see that Ananya was enamoured by his charming personality.

'By the way, doesn't she look like Riya?' Didi suddenly said.

'A little bit,' Mom grunted.

'Riya? Who?' Ananya asked.

'Don't you know? She was his girlfriend, his childhood sweetheart. I heard you both broke up?' Didi had been always sharp and cunning. Every Christmas, I had asked Santa to make her disappear.

I gave her a stern look. 'None of your business.' Yes! That was how I always talked to her.

'Gautam! Mind it! She is your elder sister,' Dad intervened.

She had spoilt the mood; the rest of the dinner was eaten in silence. I could sense Ananya's discomfort. Didi's statement had opened up a lot of questions in her mind and it would really be difficult for me to clear the cloud of doubts now. Didi was so ruthless, I hated her.

After a little chat with my mom and dad, I showed Ananya the guest room. Then I went back to talk with my parents. I told them about my life in Mumbai, omitting most of the serious stuff of course. Mom was shocked to hear about the office politics and how we were tortured. For people like my mom, life was all about shopping for jewellery and expensive saris. I discussed our business and dad was quite amazed by the progress we had made.

'All the best, son. I knew you will rock it. Nothing is unconquerable for my son,' Dad said with pride and Mom smiled. She was really happy for me and now she had a reason to celebrate. Celebration meant another chance to go shopping.

'Mom, how about Ananya?' I approached the topic apprehensively after my dad went out for some work.

'What about her?' she sensed what was coming.

'Did you like her?'

'She seems to be a very good friend of yours. Nice girl. Isn't she older than you?' she said.

I nodded, 'Four years older.'

'My goodness! Tell her to get married soon before it gets too late.' Her words actually revealed her dislike. Ananya did not share our status, she didn't belong to our caste and she wasn't younger than me. Nothing matched. *Mom says no girlfriend.*

'I will leave in an hour,' I said and stood up, showing my displeasure.

'Yeah! It's better that you drop that girl home before dark,' she said.

'Hmm...'

'But before you leave, don't forget to see your sister,' she smiled. 'You're going to be an uncle soon.'

Whoa! Didi was pregnant! Suddenly I felt that I could really forgive her for all her sins. That was the best news I had heard in a long time. It was to be the beginning of a new generation in our family; I was super excited just thinking about it. Children are actually God-sent angels who make life meaningful.

I rushed to Didi's room. She was busy talking on the phone with Jiju. She seemed happy and was blushing continuously. Pregnancy actually renewed the dead romantic side in people. Didi had always complained of Jiju being unromantic. I waited for her to finish the call. She saw me and hung up, so I went up to her and gave her a tight hug. Probably the first genuine one in all my life! I loved her for the beautiful gift she was giving our family.

'So, you talked about her to mom?' she inquired.

'How do you know?'

'I just overheard.'

I gave her a shocked look. 'You're so mean!' And we both laughed.

'So four years, huh!'

'Yeah. So? I wonder what you people are thinking. We are just going around casually.'

'It's better you both go around casually only. Don't think beyond that, it won't work.'

'C'mon, can we change the topic?'

'Hmm…'

And then it was time to return to our Mumbai adventures, this time round uncensored, except the slap gate part.

∽

'Bye Aunty, it was really nice meeting you today. Thanks for the lovely food,' Ananya said.

'The pleasure is all mine, beta,' Mom replied.

'Congratulations, Nandita!'

'Wow! He told you?' Mom quipped. 'You're very close to him. Take her home safely.'

Ananya too had realized that Mom didn't like her. Mom didn't ask a single question about her or her family; she wasn't interested in knowing her even a bit. Mom didn't even once ask her to visit again which meant that she didn't want to see Ananya again. Ananya felt insulted I knew, but I was helpless. I regretted taking her home.

We didn't talk on our return journey. To avoid looking at me, Ananya closed her eyes but I knew she was faking sleep. I tried a couple of times to break the silence between us by initiating random topics but it didn't work. I gave up trying. I drove fast and woke her up when we reached her building. She got out of the car and simply bid goodbye. I returned to my flat.

She didn't call me that night.

That Kiss in the Rain

I ran as fast as I could to reach the station by 6.07 p.m., to catch the first train after office hours. I was there two minutes early, so I walked from one end to the other of platform no. 1 and then came back to my regular spot. I missed the 6.07, then the 6.17, after that the 6.29, 6.34 and 6.46 and finally, even the 6.51 p.m. (she rarely missed the 6.51). I called her many times, but her cell was switched off. Then I tried her desk landline, someone else picked up and said that she had left long ago. She might have taken a bus or worse still, Sachin may have picked her up, I thought. But that 'switched off' recorded message on her cell was irritating me. I would go by the 7.30 fast, I decided.

One by one three more trains passed me by, but still there was no sign of her. I was worried by then. I was pacing up and down the platform in frustration when suddenly, I got a delivery report of an empty message I had sent her. I quickly dialled her number.

She cut my call.

I called again.

And again, she cut the call.

That made me furious; I hated it when anyone ignored me and that too, in such a tense situation. I hadn't heard from her after our Pune visit. So I called her again.

'What?' she screamed.

'Where were you?'

'None of your business.'

'Tell me Ananya,' I demanded.

'Uff! I was in yoga class.'

'Really?'

'Yes! Pathetic, Gautam!'

'You didn't tell me about it?'

'What do you mean by that? Why should I tell you everything?'

'Where are you now?'

'At the company gate.'

I ran out of the station and there she was, crossing the highway. She saw me and moved in another direction. I followed her, she was walking fast. I ran to close the gap and stood in front of her.

'What's wrong with you?' I asked.

'Nothing. I'm just tired. I want to go home,' she said and pushed me aside.

'OK! I want to talk to you.'

'I'm afraid that won't be possible. Look, the train is here.'

'So what? We will talk in the train.'

'No. I'm going in the ladies coach.'

'You're coming with me,' I pulled her hand.

'Gautam! Leave me or else I'll slap you,' she struggled, pulling her hand away from mine.

Of course, I didn't freak out at her words. She wasn't Moody, and more importantly, she was Ananya, she couldn't do anything. Yet I let her go because people were staring at us. The train had arrived and she quickly ran into the ladies compartment. Ten seconds later, the train had begun moving. I had hardly any time to think of anything as it accelerated and I jumped into the coach. I held the hand bar firmly and pulled myself in. And saw that I was surrounded by women.

I felt like a little mouse finding its way among a gathering of crows. I freaked out as they attacked me all at once; there was no chance of escape. They pushed me to the very edge of the foot board. I was really scared and the worst part of it all was that it was a fast train and the next stop was ten minutes away. I tried to balance myself holding on to the bar, but they went on and on and I even heard a few choice Hindi abuses like MC*** and BC*** hurled at me. Mumbai women!

There was no way out, hanging there I would've fallen down onto the tracks or hit an electric pole. I fought my way in and that irked the girls even more.

'Call the police!' 'Throw him out!' they shouted and I started to feel helpless. I looked around frantically for Ananya. There she was, sitting a few seats ahead, with her headphones on. And how pathetic was that! I cried her name out loud twice but it fell on deaf ears. And while I stood there panicking, all around me were girls who just didn't seem to stop poking and prodding me.

'Shut up!' I shouted at the top of my lungs.

It worked. They looked at me, stunned. I knew that effect would not last long and I had to do something quickly. I glanced at Ananya, she was still swaying to the music in her earphones. I ran to her, making my way through the crowd. The girls followed, oblivious to what was happening. When our eyes met, Ananya froze. It wasn't often that you found a guy in a ladies compartment.

'Gautam!' she screamed, pulling out her earphones and standing up. 'How did you get in?'

'I just jumped into the train,' I smiled.

She narrowed her eyes. 'Have you gone mad? What do you want?'

'I just want to say sorry for that day.'

'I don't know, Gautam. But I guess we should not meet anymore.'

'Have you gone mad?'

'Gautam! Please. I don't want you around.'

'What? I am not going anywhere until you promise that things will be OK between us.'

'Gautam! No. Stop messing up my life,' she was about to break into tears, that deadliest weapon girls are always ready to use.

'Throw him out! Throw him out!' the chants started again.

I gave them all a dirty look and turned back to Ananya. She felt embarrassed; she sat on her seat and started crying, covering her face in her palms. I wondered what the big deal was. Anyway, crying was what girls did for timepass. They could shed them at will and touch everyone's heart.

We guys too have our weapon, that little sheepish smile and an expression of utter childlike innocence. It didn't work all the time though. I was afraid I would be thrown out of the train right then, but that happened to be my lucky day.

'Hey!' one young girl quipped, 'I don't know what your problem is but it's something related to love.' Now it wasn't about an intruder in their territory anymore, it was getting filmy and romantic and they were enjoying it.

'And he is so cute!'

'Thank you,' I blushed but Ananya wasn't impressed. She stood up and put her hands on her hip and gave me a cold stare.

'Girl! You're crazy! Look, he loves you so much,' another voice chimed in. My smile widened, my victory was on its way.

'Shut up! You all know nothing,' Ananya yelled at them.

'Maybe he made some mistake but he is apologizing. You should forgive him.' It just kept coming. I was loving it. Who said there was no humanity in the world?

'What do you want me to do then?' Ananya was dazed, 'forgive him and hug him?!'

'Yes! Hug him!' they all said in chorus.

I never thought that it could get that much better; I looked at Ananya for her reaction. She seemed lost and I was on cloud nine.

'Hug him!' the public demand was even louder now.

I wondered what was actually going on in her mind. She gave me a strange look, one that made me think that a slap, not a hug, seemed a distinct possibility. But as I said, it was my lucky day and there came our first official romantic hug.

She put her arms around me and held me tight. I could feel her heart beat; it was racing and so was mine. I wasn't really prepared for the hug and the presence of the crowd made it difficult, though I owed this one to them. I closed my eyes with a feeling of awkwardness and thought about how it would end and what would come after. I left it to Ananya, I could still hear the cheers and roars throughout the compartment.

∽

We had sunk Samir's project; we offered Mr Bose such a tempting deal that he could not possibly refuse it. It was a sort of loss for us, but money had never been our priority; we only wanted to see Samir down on his knees. Finally, we were to get our revenge. We delivered the assignment in record time and Samir was sacked from his job on the pretext of downsizing the bench, citing the recession.

I was now relaxed, I could finally sleep in peace and I did just that. It was like a period of hibernation for me. For two days, I locked myself in my room, switched off my cell and had no contact with the world—*sirf main aur meri tanhaiye.* That's when I started to think about my future beyond this IT life. In a way, I had achieved what I had wanted from my move to Mumbai. I had a job, great friends and a booming business. The important thing was that I was independent now; I didn't need my dad's name to survive. So what next, I thought. Should I call Riya and tell her everything? I knew I had done everything I could to get her back but she never responded. There was no point waiting for her anymore, she was gone forever, I concluded. She was seeing some NRI guy there, I had found out from a few common friends. She was a closed chapter and I had moved on. I decided I could now pack my bags and return home to enjoy the rest of my life. But what about Ananya? She had never loved me, she loved Sachin. But was I ready to lose her to that ugly idiot. Being with Ananya was always a game with new pieces added now and then for twists and thrills.

I remembered her last message after our train hug: *I don wan u 2 xpect nything aftr this hug. U knw it was a 4ced 1.*

I had been too busy to reply. The next day had been 1 June, her birthday. I had something planned for her—girls loved surprises.

I left the office early that day and went shopping. There were lot of preparations to be made. I had to order a cake, get a gift and I had very little time in hand. I wanted to make this birthday very special to her. She had told me once that her birthday was never celebrated like my birthday might have been celebrated. Undoubtedly, I agreed. My birthday bashes were always stupendous. Dad had once invited SRK and that was actually the first time that SRK had visited Pune. The news had been splashed everywhere across the papers and TV. Anyway, I had other ideas for Ananya.

'Can I have a Barbie doll please?' I asked at a toy shop.

The lady asked me, 'What's the age of the girl?'

'Well, she is twenty-eight. Actually, she is turning twenty-nine today,' I said sheepishly.

The lady gave me a blank look.

∞

So at 11.55 p.m., I was outside her building. Everything was ready. It was showtime. I climbed the stairs and stood at her front door, wondering whether I should go in. The house seemed quiet, even the light was dim. Were they sleeping? What would her mother think? And what would Ananya herself think of it? It was midnight and if I was expecting a warm welcome, then I was stupid. I didn't want to spoil her birthday, so I hung the cake and gift on her doorknob. I rang the bell and ran down the stairs as fast as I could.

I got a call from Ananya.

'Gautam, thank you!' she giggled.

'For what?' I pretended to be ignorant.

'As if you don't know.'

'What are you talking about?'

'So you seriously don't know? Then, I guess Sachin did it. He is so romantic,' she was very smart.

'Shut up! Ananya, it's me who left those gifts there, OK!'

'Really? Where are you then?'

'In the parking lot of your building.'

'Thank you! But sorry, I can't call you upstairs. Mom is sleeping.'

'Okay! I understand. Then you come down.'

'Are you mad? I have to change for that. I am in a nightie.'

'Wow! I missed it.'

'Shut up! Anyway you didn't wish me even once yet.'

'Wait Ma'am, I am not done yet.'

'What more do you have for me?' she sounded excited. I could hear her, unwrapping the gift.

'Gautam! It's a Barbie doll!'

'You always wanted to have one, right?'

'As a child. Not now,' she cleared.

'It doesn't matter. I will give you everything that you want.'

'That's so sweet, thank you!'

'Hmmm…'

'The cake is awesome too.'

'Your favourite black forest from your favourite Monginis.'

'Oh! Somebody is doing quite a lot of research on me,' she teased.

'I can do anything for you.'

'Boss! You're such a drameybaaz.'

'Hey! Enough now come to the balcony. I've got something for you.'

'What?' she inquired. I could hear her run through the room.

And when she came out on her balcony, she was just bamboozled. There were hundreds of candles arranged in a cluster on the ground, forming the words 'Happy Birthday' in the playground right next to her building. We were still on the phone.

'God! Gautam! How did you do that?'

'It's magic. Magic candles actually, which don't get extinguished easily.'

'Very funny,' she blushed. 'Wait, I'm coming there.'

In a moment, I saw her running towards me. She didn't change, she was in a nightie, a loose one. I could do nothing but gape at her with a wide open mouth as the testosterone levels in my bloodstream shot up.

'So, it's my lucky day.'

'Shut up, Gautam and stop staring at me like that.'

'Gosh! You look so hot.'

'I am going.'

'Wait! Ananya! Don't go,' I held her hand. I didn't want her to go anywhere, I wanted her to stay with me like that forever.

Was it just a wonderful coincidence or our chemistry that the rain seemed to witness our romance every time we were together in a moment like that? The wind blew hard and took away all the magic from the candles as one by one, they all went down. I looked at the sky; the stars were already hidden behind a thick blanket of cloud. The monsoons had arrived.

I remembered a line from a greeting card. *The day you were born, it was raining hard. Actually, the sky was crying because the most beautiful star had fallen to earth.* So apt for Ananya. Perhaps, the sky mourned every year on her birthday.

There was the roar of thunder then which brought Ananya closer to me. She stood clutching my arm. She was scared but she felt safe with me. The atmosphere was romantic enough to freeze anyone's feet. The rain was to follow, we realized, as a few droplets fell on our arms. We tried to move fast towards a tree but the rain gave us competition. We stopped at the gate to the playground, standing under a tree for a shelter as it started raining heavily. I looked at her; she looked so gorgeous in the rain, the droplets from her hair making their way in little streams down her face. I stopped them with my hand at her nose.

'What?' she stared.

'I won't let the rain kiss you before me.'

And I kissed her. We kissed.

Love, a Rather Bad Idea!

That kiss had changed the entire equation. It wasn't a game anymore. I desired her, I needed her. I couldn't sleep all night after I got home that day. I texted her immediately that I had reached. She didn't reply. I checked the time; it was 3.00 in the morning. She was asleep definitely but I wanted to wait for her message even if it meant waiting for an eternity.

'Good morning, Gautam,' Ananya's call woke me up in the morning.

'Hello Anu…' I said in a sleepy voice. I didn't know when I had dozed off; I hadn't changed my clothes and was lying on the couch. I had been thinking and dreaming about her all night.

'Gautam, wake up! It's already nine,' she said.

'Is it? Ananya, I don't want to go to office today. Let's go somewhere and celebrate your birthday.'

'We already did that, right?'

'OK! Then see you at lunch.'

'No. Gautam, I won't come to office today. I've got to meet a few relatives today. I will call you later. OK. Bye.'

'Bye.'

I carried my drowsiness to the office. I moved around at the speed of a snail, I just didn't want to work that day. I was late as always but didn't care about it. At the most they would throw me out, I thought, and anyway, I had stopped giving a damn about my fucking job. I now had options beyond it. I was a successful entrepreneur.

I waited for her to call all day but she didn't. At first, I took it casually but by afternoon, I started missing her. Many times through the day, I thought of calling her but I didn't want to disturb her when she was with her family. But when she hadn't called me even after office hours, I started to worry. I was still not sure whether I should call her, I didn't dare to upset her on her birthday. Ultimately, I gave in to temptation and dialled her number.

She didn't pick up and I called her again. There was no response and then I got the message that her phone was switched off. My worries only worsened. I grew extremely restless and finished almost a full packet of cigarettes in frustration. I didn't know why I was overreacting so much, it wasn't the first time that she hadn't taken my calls. Yet something was bothering me and I had to act on it.

I drove to her house and almost ran up the stairs. But when I reached her door, I felt acutely embarrassed. I saw a lot of shoes outside her flat and could hear the loud chaos within which only meant that she was fine. I had this urge to ring the bell and probably join them all but was I invited? *No.* I smiled thinking about it and was about to trace back my steps when unfortunately, the door opened. My greatest fear turned into reality; it was Sachin standing in front of me.

'Hey! You're Ananya's colleague, right?' he said with a big grin. I wanted to break his teeth. I gave him a forced smile.

'Come in! Come in! Dude, it's her birthday.' And he pulled me in.

'Ananya! Look who is here,' he went in to call her. I was now in the middle of a few freaky kids and curious oldies, all staring at me. I guessed they didn't appreciate my visit. All I could do was stand there and smile at them foolishly.

'Come here,' he was pulling Ananya out, holding her hand. I wanted to break his hands.

Ananya too didn't seem happy to see me. It was far more than shock that I saw in her eyes. She stood so still, staring at me like she was dead. At least, I desperately wished she was. How could she do this? What kind of a girl was she? What did she really want? The questions kept coming in my mind and my hatred grew even more. Looking at us both, I felt that Sachin understood something of what was going on between us, and if he didn't, then he was a chimpanzee for sure. No, wait! Chimpanzees are intelligent!

'Hey! What happened?' he shook her shoulder.

'Nothing,' her lips twitched as she tried to pretend that everything was normal.

'Hey! Gautam right?' he still acted like a jerk. 'I talked to her mom, we are getting married soon.'

That crushed me. Ananya too seemed astonished, maybe because he spilled the beans without her permission. He hugged her. Of course, I wanted to break his ribs. *But why him?* I was the one who was stupid. I had known everything and yet I had fallen for it. I should rather break my own head, I thought.

'Congratulations, buddy! Happy for you both,' I wished them. Ananya looked down at her feet.

'I must leave now. I am in a hurry.' Saying this I got out of there. I was suffocating within.

∾

I knew she would definitely call me; I was eagerly waiting for it. I was prepared for it. I had been drinking ever since I had returned from her house but I didn't feel a bit of drowsiness; nothing could have doused my spirits. I wasn't upset or depressed. I was furious and I had made up my mind—if she tried to play any more games with me, then God save her.

It was nearing midnight when the long wait for her call ended. I picked up immediately.

'Ananya! I give it to you. You start. I want to hear it all, tell me why?' I blasted.

She started to cry, I had expected that. I was not going to melt though.

'Stop this drama. Just shoot.'

'I just want to say, I'm sorry for everything I did to you. I am so mean and selfish.'

'You think you can escape by saying all that. I'm gonna ruin you forever.'

'I do deserve a punishment,' she wept. 'I wish we had never met. Please, go away from my life.'

'How can you even say that? Just twenty-four hours ago, you kissed me.'

'That was actually the biggest mistake of my life. The truth is that I love Sachin.'

I wondered what substance this girl was made of.

'Do you even have a heart to love someone?'

'Yes! I'm heartless. I'm a slut. Fine? Are you happy with it?'

So after doing all that she had done, she still had the guts to give me attitude. I wanted to slap her right then. Only that would relieve me from this frustration, I felt.

'I want to meet you.'

'No. Gauti, I don't want to see you again in my life. Forget me and move on. Forgive me, if you can.' She hung up.

The conversation had not turned out anywhere close to what I had planned. Perhaps, it wasn't I who had the last laugh. She did it to me again; she had called me to insult me. That thought drove me mad; I first flung the phone down on the floor and then, a vase from the table. I was in a breaking spree and nobody was there to stop me. I looked at the TV. A cricket match was on. God of cricket was batting. I read his name. It hurt. I hate all the Sachins in this world, I said aloud and broke the TV too. I wanted to break everything that came my way, maybe breaking down the whole little world I had built around me would give me some solace, I thought. Because my heart was now broken mercilessly, not once but twice.

∾

When I woke up, I realized I was in a hospital. Richa was sitting beside me. She told me that Subho and Pritam had visited me when I didn't show up at the office and hadn't received any calls after that night. The doctors had said that I was unconscious due to excess drinking. I had fallen on the ground at home, unconscious, she explained. Though it wasn't anything serious to worry about, I was advised to control my drinking habits. Whatever! My only concern was to get out of that sick place. I hated being in hospital—the boring atmosphere, that constant bloody stench, those white curtains and sheets, continuous beeps sounding from various equipments, stale and tasteless food, the dull faces of the doctors, crying patients and no TV or internet—all these were enough to make any healthy person sick. I felt a phobia rising in my mind that I would never get well staying in that hospital. I grew restless and insisted on going back home.

I was discharged in the evening but the formalities were an uphill task. I tell you, I had not done so much paper work even in my college days. Those numerous forms made me feel that I was being released from a jail and not from a hospital. But I had a loud mouth in Richa, things got done rather easily. *Aise har ek friend zaroori hota hai!* So true.

'Hey Gautam, look! Moody is here too!' Subho had found the name in a register not meant for our eyes.

'What?'

'See, her name is written here,' he showed us the entry.

'There can be many people in the city with that name.'

'Boss! See carefully, the surname is also the same,' he now placed the register on my lap.

It read Mudrika Kodigre.

'Not a big deal. Many people do have the same name and surname,' I said but I wasn't sure by then. She would never have thought I would visit the same hospital. Perhaps, the entry being made in the maternity care section had got us more interested. Maybe she was there to visit someone else admitted in the maternity ward; we all hoped that was the truth. Richa went on to ask the receptionist about it and found out that Moody had an appointment with the doctor the previous day and had another one on that very day.

We waited impatiently outside the hospital to know the truth and after a wait of more than one hour, finally, she showed up. She was alone and seemed disturbed. She headed straight to the maternity ward after checking with the receptionist. We tried to get some details from the receptionist but she refused to share any information which led to another two hours of waiting.

Finally, she came out. She looked different, she seemed to have grown weak and thin. She had dark circles around her eyes, her skin had lost its colour. She dragged her feet to the taxi stand, holding a polythene bag with a bunch of papers in it. There were tear stains running down her cheeks, she seemed to have cried a lot. Well, connecting each dot of this mystery only led to one conclusion.

Moody was pregnant.

Richa stopped her on the road. Seeing her, Moody burst into tears and fell into her arms. Richa helped her get in the car and I drove us all to my house. She cried hard all the way, as both Richa and Subho tried to console her. The child was gone, she told them. That came as a shock to us; no one knew how to react to that. You only heard these things in Bollywood movies but this was real. She had become pregnant and had just aborted the little life. Wasn't that a crime? OK, not legally but ethically.

We guessed the rest of the story. Samir had ditched her after being sacked and had run to the US. Their morning romance had resulted in this child but her condition was taboo in our society. And the baby was killed even before it could see the sunrise. So who was to be blamed for this murder, Moody? Samir? Our society? Or Masti IT Solutions? After all, we had played a major part in getting Samir fired from his job. I had never felt guiltier.

'Stupid! How can you be so careless?' Richa scolded Moody.

'It just happened. We love each other.'

'Really? Where is he now then?' Subho joined in.

'He is in the US to get a job. He will be back soon.'

'If so, then why did you have to go for an abortion?' Richa argued.

Moody broke into tears once again, 'I was alone. I was scared.'

'Yes! You're alone. He has run away forever. He is such a pervert and coward.' Both of them went gaga over it, I watched them from a distance. I still hadn't forgotten that slap.

'No. He will come back. It wasn't his fault exactly. He lost his job to outsourcing,' she defended him.

We all looked at each other. There was Moody, one of our major enemies crying after a big setback in life and somewhere, we had played a hand in things leading up to it. We had achieved our goal, but at what cost? Destroying one life and taking another. I felt so ashamed of myself. I felt a big lump in my throat. *I was now a murderer! A bloody murderer!*

'Moody, that outsourcing company belongs to me,' I confessed.

She looked at me immediately, her eyes blazing with fury. She reached out for me savagely but Richa came in between us.

'It's not just him. We all own it together,' Richa said.

'What?' She was stunned to hear that. Her feet trembled in shock and she sat on the couch with her hands on her head. She was crying again. Louder.

'You're scoundrels. You ruined my life.'

'Shut up. It's you who ruined it. Bloody fool,' Richa swore.

Moody paused and looked at Richa.

'Yes, Moody. Don't you still see Samir is bad?'

'What do you mean?'

'Did he call you even once?'

She shook her head, 'He must be busy.'

'Whom are you kidding Moody? You also know well that he is gone. He won't come back. And anyway, it's not our fault at all. He was to go to the US and leave you anyway. We just made it happen earlier.'

'No. No...' Moody bawled. 'He will come back. I know. I know.'

She never really accepted the truth. She continued to believe that he would be back, but he didn't. He didn't even call her and yet she kept waiting. It was actually hard to say why she was so adamant, was it really her love for him or her *I-am-always-right* ego? We never found out but we saw her breaking down a bit every day. She had forgiven us but had turned completely numb by then. We tried hard, giving our best to retrieve our bubbly Moody but she was lost somewhere in the dark memories of her love.

Love...a rather bad idea!

Everything You Desire

*I*t was Ali's idea. He had made the proposal and mailed it to the party in the US. The party, a research lab in New York, had shown interest and wanted to meet us. They were working on some hardware which would project a 3D image of people involved in video chat and they wanted us to handle the software involved. They were keen on getting the deal done as soon as possible and asked us to have our passports and other documents ready so that they could send us the air tickets.

'Ali, how could you do this without even asking us?' I questioned him and the others were equally furious about it.

'What's wrong in this? It's just another project for Masti IT Solutions. Why are you guys overreacting?' he justified.

'We have had enough of that shit. Don't you know exactly what happened because of it? It's over now,' I said.

'Damn! At least you don't talk like that, Gautam. It has got nothing to do with Moody.'

We all glared at him and he stopped blabbering. Moody stayed out of it, she was sitting in one corner of the room. But she had heard it all. So another emotional fiasco was a certainty. We were seriously fed up of putting up with Moody; every time something like that happened, she would moan for some time and make us feel guilty for a few days. *Ali! You suck.*

'Let me see it,' she rose from her seat to have a look at the mail. She read it carefully while we waited for her reaction. I truly prayed that she would slap me instead of sobbing for the rest of the day.

She finished reading it and stretched out her arms comfortably, apparently thinking about something, while we waited with bated breath. 'Can I join your company?'

That was indeed a shocker. We all looked at each other stunned and then shouted out in joy. Richa ran to hug Moody. That smile on Moody's face had taken such a long time coming. It was celebration time; Pritam was already on his way to the wine shop. Black Dog Premium! It was a really big occasion. In fact, big is an understatement. It was huge!

'They have even agreed to send us an advance of one million dollars,' Ali announced.

'Gosh! That's almost five crores,' Subho exclaimed. 'Eighty lakhs each. We're finally gonna be rich!'

That little calculation set our spirits soaring. The advance amount each one of us was to receive was almost equivalent to the sum of everyone's annual package at our company multiplied by three, and that was just the beginning. Big money was to follow. We had hit a jackpot. Just thinking about the prospects gave me tingles in my stomach. I looked at Moody, the pretty smile was still there, but I knew it wasn't about the money. For her, it was actually about the trip to the US. *Mr Samir, we're coming!*

∽

The annual day of our company was celebrated every year on the founder's birthday and it was always a stupendous event. A week-long celebration, with various competitions like painting, photography, fashion shows, dances, skits and singing. There were sports too—cricket tournaments, football matches, badminton, carrom, scrabble and chess. They all seemed out of my league but participation in at least one event was mandatory for all youngsters and I didn't want to join the league of non-participant uncles.

'So, what about you guys?' We were discussing the fest.

'Well, Pritam is in the cricket and football teams; Richa and Moody are participating in painting; Ali has enrolled in photography and I'll be rocking the ramp,' Subho proudly declared. Subho was obsessed with fashion shows. His Facebook profile was full of numerous photos of him walking the ramp. He genuinely thought he had the charm and attitude to make the difference but that little paunch of his spoiled everything. Yet he would always be the first person to show up for auditions.

'I think I will go for chess,' I said.

'What? Dude! You need to have a brain for that,' Subho cracked one of his poor jokes but the others still laughed.

'Hey! They say they will have a boxing tournament this time,' Ali said.

'That's great. I can try that then,' I said.

'What? C'mon, I was kidding that you don't have a brain. Why are you taking it seriously?' Subho laughed.

Well, they didn't know yet that I was once called the Mike Tyson of my college.

After lunch, I went to the health club for registration. They told me that they hadn't got a single entry yet for the tournament. I wondered whether I was to win it without even fighting. But boxing was something I had always taken seriously. It's not a sport that you can decide to try on impulse and jump into the ring, you will be knocked out in no time. Boxing needs serious practice and I had two weeks in hand. Though that wasn't really enough, I was confident.

Later that day, I took out my boxing gloves and the punching bag. I called my friends to help me set it up. We filled the punching bag with sand and hung it from the ceiling of my drawing room. Over the next few days, I exercised hard in the gym, in the mornings, to regain my fitness levels and practiced again at night till I fell on my knees. My friends would often visit me and see me dedicatedly working at it but they still didn't take me seriously and mocked me.

'If by wearing gloves, you can become a boxer, then I own a guitar, I should be a rock star,' Subho teased me. I didn't mind, I didn't feel like arguing with them. The big day was nearing and I was ready for the challenge.

Boxing was something new to the people in my company and it attracted a lot of attention. People seemed excited about a boxing match and gathered to watch in good numbers, but the same enthusiasm seemed missing when it came to participation. Apart from me, there was only one other entry and I was sure it must be some soft bodied wannabe from the gym.

Winning it looked like a piece of cake to me; one good punch in the right area and I would be the champ. I roared at the audience as I stepped into the ring, a big applause followed and my opponent walked in. Gajendra Verma, the commentator announced. I couldn't believe my ears. I turned around and was astounded to see that loser from Ananya's group coming up to the ring. I looked around the audience and found her. She was there with her friends, sitting in a corner. Just as she had not known about my dad, this boxing thing too had been kept a secret. Of course, like my friends, she too had thought I was too cute for the game. Anyway, I had for an opponent a guy whom I had always wanted to hit, so now was my big chance to do it in front of a big crowd and be applauded, honoured and prized for it.

With the bell, the match started. If I had thought Gajendra to be naïve, I was absolutely right. He didn't even know how to throw a punch right. Having a good gym-toned body and imitating the moves from the movie *Rocky* were not going to make any difference. I soon tired of his stupid jigs and wanted to end the match as soon as possible. I couldn't stand the sight of him. He wore large headgear that protected him but my hard punches would have been enough to give him a concussion. However, I wanted to end it in a style, with a single punch showdown. A straight jab on his chin would actually do the trick but Gajendra had learnt something from Sylvester Stallone after all. He covered his face well and I had to wait for my chance. I attacked from all directions but he was solid in his defense. I tried even harder but that made me tired and affected my concentration. I became a little casual about it and started to loosen up. Gajendra saw that as a ripe opportunity and pounced over me to surprise me with a few quick punches. His punches didn't really hurt me as much as Ananya's loud cheers did. I used my experience to get back my control over the game and hit him hard. Ananya frowned. I wondered what her intention was—was she supporting Gajendra's win or my defeat. The thought disturbed me but somewhere deep inside, I knew that she still cared for me. And I wanted to prove it.

After surprising him with a few hooks, I stood still in front of him, staring in her direction. Gajendra was puzzled at my action but he eventually guessed my motive and threw a hard punch at my stomach. Stupid lout! Didn't even know that there were no points to gain from hitting in the stomach. Ananya was unfazed. She wanted to walk away but her friends held her back. They wanted to see the match to the finish. Gajendra hit me on my chest but he still couldn't even move me. I roared aloud right in his face, shaking him up a bit and that excited the crowd into cheering and calling my name out loud. I was turning into a hero. I gave Ananya a look but she simply looked away. Gajendra gathered courage and hooked me in my ears and that really hurt. When I didn't respond, he grew confident and attacked me with a flurry of punches all over my face. I was pushed, dragged and chased all over the ring; I was literally being strangled by him. My face tore in places and blood gushed out. My friends decided that was enough and ran up to the referee to stop the match but I signalled that I was fine. And then came a strong jab, straight at my nose and I tumbled to the floor. The crowd booed my fall, I had become their favourite. Lying on the floor, I struggled to breathe, my body slowly seemed to be giving up. My vision was blurred as I tried to search Ananya in the crowd. She was still there but I saw that she now had tears in her eyes. Those beautiful eyes spoke everything she wanted to tell me. She ran forward and stood at the edge of the ring. The referee started to count.

'Why are you doing this?' she asked.

'Just want to know whether you care or not,' I mumbled. Seven seconds to go.

She frowned. 'Are you mad?' Five.

'Just say it once. Please.' Three.

'I do. OK!' One.

It happened in a flash; I rose and hit him hard in the mouth. He didn't make a sound. All I saw was him falling on the ground with his eyes wide open in shock. He only came to his senses the next day, I was later informed. He had a broken jaw with two teeth gone and it took him about two months to recover physically. As for recovering mentally…I can't say!

∽

My wounds were deep too and I had to be admitted to a hospital for a couple of days. I had become a hero after that match and everybody visited me. I was very pleased with the attention I got. And the big moment came when Ananya visited me.

'Gauti!' she sounded quite filmy. *Will she run to me and hug me?*

'Anu!' I smiled. 'Ouch!' It hurt even to smile.

'See what you have done to yourself?'

'I don't know about me but I did a lot of damage to your friend.'

'Whatever. That was really pathetic!'

'See Ananya, why don't you just accept that you care for me?'

She frowned, 'I don't.'

'Then why are you here?'

'You're so impossible.'

'Is it me Ananya? It's like you made me walk right into your heart and I did so blindly, carelessly, and finally, when I lost my way, you wanted me to get out,' I said. I knew I sounded filmy like Subho. *Sangat ka asar.*

'What do you mean by that? Did I ask you to fall in love with me?'

'But you did ask me whether I do or not which actually made me realize that I do, and then all this followed. It is your fault.'

'OK then, I'm sorry. That was a mistake.'

'A sorry won't do it. It's your fault and why should I suffer?'

'What do you want?'

'You.'

'Gauti, try to understand. I am with Sachin.'

'And what about me?' I stared at her for a long while demanding an answer but she couldn't utter a word.

'I have to go. Bye now,' she said simply and ran away.

Her behaviour spoilt my mood for the rest of that day; I wanted to be alone after that. I wanted to mourn again. Nothing was working out for me and I couldn't understand what went on in her mind. It seemed the best idea to move on from her, but I realized I was too much in love with her. I wondered that day whether I had actually thought of getting my revenge at Riya by ruining Ananya. But in the end, it was Ananya who was ruining me.

'It has turned out a lot more complicated than I ever thought it would,' my love guru Ali said.

'So what now?' I asked.

'Tell me what do you actually want.'

I shook my head, 'I don't know.'

'Well then, I will just say this much. Fuck a girl and she will love you. Love a girl and she will fuck you.'

∽

It took me a week to persuade Ananya to agree to a last dinner with me. She relented but insisted that I should not take it as a date. I had to nod but I had a plan in my mind. A stupid one.

'Hi!' she greeted me cheerfully.

'Hello!' I smiled.

'I have to get back home before 9.30.'

'Ananya! You haven't got in the car yet and you want to go.'

'Ummm…' She hesitated a bit and then got in.

I drove to Ice and Spice in Seawoods. It was the only place that had a disco and a good restaurant and was also near my place. My plan was going well so far, I thought. The stupid plan.

Dinner was great; I had used every trick in the book to make it a perfect date. A candle-lit corner table, amazing cuisines to sample from, decorations all over the place and light music, which was always a turn on for girls. It's weird how girls expect a table full of dishes though they know they are going to taste just a pinch of it all, but they will still make a hole in the pocket. Anyway, she was really amused by my royal treat and she didn't resist when I held her hand. As per plan, I ordered wine.

'What's this?' she made a face.

'Wine,' I said sheepishly.

'You know I don't drink.'

'C'mon, nothing will happen with a sip.'

'Still. I mean, you only told me not drink when you're out with a guy.'

'Oye! I said that for Gajendra. You're comparing me with him? Seriously, you spoilt the evening,' I turned my face away.

'Sorry Gautam! I didn't mean it.'

'Whatever. I will drink alone.' I took a glass and started pouring the wine making an irritating gurgling sound.

'Will you stop it?'

'Stop what?'

'Pathetic! OK! I will just have a little.'

I happily made a drink for her, this time without any special effects. She picked up her glass and tapped my glass excitedly; it was her first drink. She took a sip and almost immediately spilled it.

'Ughh! It tastes like phenyl.'

'What?'

'Yes.'

'Anu! Take it steadily. Try to feel its aroma.'

She gave it a second try and after a few hiccups, she finished her glass.

'How was it?' I watched her curiously.

'I want to puke.'

'Yuck!'

'Kidding! Can I have one more?'

'Sure.'

And it just went on and on. She had the same expression after every finished glass, as if she wanted to puke. But luckily, she didn't. She blabbered a lot of rubbish instead. She talked about everything right from her first school, her first crush, her first date, all of which I had heard a lot of times before. Girls actually don't need to drink to talk rubbish. She had set an alarm in her phone which rang at 9.30 but she was not even in a state to cancel it.

'Gautam! You idiot! How will I go home?'

'Don't worry, it's a regular thing for me. I will drive you safely.'

'And what will I tell my mom?'

I pretended to be worried. 'Then?'

'Can I stay at your place tonight?' she asked.

I faked concern again. 'Yes. But…' I said reluctantly.

'Don't worry, I always carry my toothbrush in my bag.'

I wondered how many such night-outs she had done before.

'But what about your mom?'

'Well, I will call her and say that I'm staying back at Sana's place.'

'Are you sure you can talk to her?'

'What do you mean? I'm fine. You just stay here. I don't want Mom to know that I'm with a guy.'

She went to the washroom so that she could talk to her mom without the sound of music in the background. I was worried, I had completely forgotten to plan for this part of the scenario. However, she came out smiling. I hoped that she had handled it well. I helped her out of the restaurant and drove her back to my place.

'Boss! You stay here?' she asked, her words slurring. We were still in the car, outside my apartment. She was leaning heavily on my shoulder.

I nodded.

'You're a really rich man!'

I gave her a smile and said, 'Then marry me.'

'Shut up, Gautam! That won't happen. Even you know it, so stop bothering me about it.'

'Just because I'm four years younger. I'm rich.'

'Yeah! All of that and also Riya?'

'What about her?'

'You love her and not me.'

'It's not like that Anu.'

'I've seen this world more than you. I know exactly what you wanted. You just wanted to fill the emptiness of your life with me, right?'

I turned away.

'C'mon, it's not just you, even I used you. I wanted to make Sachin feel my presence in his life and it worked. He has proposed to me,' she said. My heart broke into a million pieces.

Now I really didn't want her around. The plan was totally stupid, I thought. But she had to spend the night at my place and I didn't know how I would bear it. She just went on and on with stories of her romance with that ugly pig. Spending the night in my car or in the lift seemed a better idea.

'Gauti, wait. Where are you going?'

I didn't pay attention and got out of the car. She came running and trudged alongside me.

'Stop! It's not safe outside. You're drunk.'

I mocked her. 'Look who is talking.'

'Oh c'mon! It was you who made me drink. So, now that I'm drunk, instead of taking advantage of me, you're walking away.'

'What?' I was amused to hear that.

'Yes! I'm helpless. You can do anything. Go for the kill,' she said innocently. And that had actually been my brilliant plan, going by Ali's mantra. I now felt ashamed of myself for stooping so low.

Ananya was helpless indeed. I carried her to my bedroom and put her down on the bed. The alcohol had already taken its toll, she dozed off. She shivered a little and held me tighter. I took a blanket and covered her. I sat on a chair next to the bed, watching her sleep.

That night, I didn't close my eyes even once.

T(w)o 'States'

I would call it a magical night because it changed my life forever. Sitting on the chair, I kept looking at her. The chilly breeze made me shiver but I couldn't afford to go to another room to get my jacket or even get up to look in the cupboard for another blanket. It was that amazing to just watch her sleep. My room had a sun roof which always helped me wake up in the mornings but that night, I understood its real meaning. As the night wore on, the moon rose and shone brighter with every passing moment. It was as if moonlight was being absorbed into my room; all the lights were off and yet my room was brightly lit. Her face shone like a halo and I wondered what she was dreaming of as she smiled in her sleep. The fragrance of her skin enveloped me. I fell in love with her more and more with every beat of my heart that night.

Night turned into day and the birds started chirping with the first rays of the sun. Slowly, the sun grew brighter and shone his rays right into my room, through the sun roof. It disturbed her and she tossed and turned to fight the flooding light. I was so mesmerized that I sat staring at her beautiful face instead of reaching up to cover the sun roof.

'Umm...' she made a face like an innocent child and stretched. Yawning, she sat up in bed.

She was now wide awake. She looked around and realized that it was not her house. She saw me, and in a moment, recalled everything from last night. Seeing her expression, I couldn't make out what she was thinking but I was freaked out about what her reaction would be.

'We didn't do anything right, last night?'

I pacified her. She narrowed her eyes. She was angry.

'I want to go home,' she got up and started gathering her stuff.

'Fine. I will drop you home.'

'Just stay away from me,' she said.

With wet eyes she stormed out of my flat. Was she upset? Or was she angry?

I dialled her number but cut the call instantly even before the first ring. I was scared of her anger. Moreover, I felt that there was no point in staying at home and thinking about it all day. I would only feel miserable and end up doing something stupid. So I drove to the office.

∾

'Gosh! Look at you, didn't you sleep last night?' Moody inquired. We were at the food court for breakfast. I was dying to share the story but I didn't want to complicate the situation further.

'Guys! I've got great news for you,' Ali joined us and threw a sheet of paper on the table. Moody grabbed it and began to read. I noticed a few words and knew it was a letter from the States.

She finished reading while the rest of us waited for the announcement. 'We did it,' she screamed.

'Are you sure?' Richa snatched the paper from her and read. She too gave the same reaction.

We had finally made it. Wow, it felt great. We congratulated each other and then huddled together in a hug.

'We're leaving next week. They have even sent the advance,' Ali showed us the cheque.

We deposited it immediately in our company account and by noon, we got the SMS that the amount was credited to our account. We had become rich.

We got busy with the coding of the pilot programme so that we could make a good impression in the minds of the Americans before we hit their shores. We dreamt of becoming the next Steve Jobs. The project was to be the next big thing in the IT world; it was to bring about a new revolution in the development of science and technology. If Skype was the best thing that had happened to distant relationships, this was even bigger. Parents would never feel the absence of their children staying abroad. Relationships would never die in the pretext of distance. Distance would now only be a word.

'So what have you decided?' Subho asked me.

'What's there to decide, we are surely going to the States? Nothing's gonna stop us.'

'But we have a bond with the company.'

'So, we will pay the bond amount and get ourselves freed out of here,' I suggested.

'What? That's a lot of money,' Subho protested.

'Ya, but in a way, this amount does belong to the company. We cheated it. And the experience letter from here would really prove handy,' I explained and everyone agreed.

So, we decided to put in our papers that very day so that we could devote more time to the new project. Typing the resignation letter is actually the best feeling in an IT company. It marks your freedom from slavery until your joining date with another company where you will go back to selling yourself again for some extra bucks. This is what implies growth in the corporate world where emotion or attachment has no value. Life here simply rocks, I tell you.

Subho spent the whole day typing the resignation letter and then the letter bidding adieu to other colleagues. Everyone else copied his letters merrily but I had other plans. I still hated Muthu the pig and was in no mood to move on gracefully. But I didn't have the time to write something original either, after completing those long-drawn formalities of resignation. They had even more rituals than a South Indian wedding! I ended up writing the shortest and most expressive letter to Muthu. My letter simply read: FUCK OFF.

❧

Ding dong, my door bell rang.

'Let me get it,' Richa ran to the door, 'Must be the pizza boy.'

That was to be our last meal in India before we left for the US in the evening. We had gathered at my place for the last day, just to make sure that we left together and nothing went wrong. We ended up partying and having a great time. Life is never fun without some awesome friends.

'Gautam!' she called out, 'Please come here.'

'C'mon Richa! You pay the bill,' I shouted from my room.

'I asked you to come here.' That was a straight threat. I ran out to check.

OMG! Ananya? What she was doing there? I had not heard from her since that night. A lot of other things had gone right after that day and I realized that I needed to move on to better things in life than just chasing girls. Coding languages had helped me forget that I was in love with the girl standing at the door. But looking at her then, I wondered whether I had really moved on. I told myself I had, since I had been thinking of nothing but becoming the next Steve Jobs or Mark Zuckerberg for so many days. What did she want now, I wanted to know. I was going away from her life forever.

'Gauti...' she said.

'Hi!' I smiled.

'Where are you these days? I don't see you in the office anywhere. Your number is not reachable. So I called your landline and they said you had resigned. What's going on?'

'Well, it's a long story...' I shrugged. 'Tell me, what's up?'

'I want to talk to you.'

'Yeah! Tell me.'

She looked around at the others who had gathered near the door. 'Alone,' she said and the others turned to go back in.

'Wait. It's OK, Ananya. They are my friends, you can speak in front of them.'

'Still, I insist.'

I shook my head and looked at Richa. She was staring at me furiously. Nobody messes with her, I remembered, so I took Ananya to my room and the others waited outside.

'What?' I asked.

'I don't know what to say, Gauti. I just missed you a lot.'

Uff! Irritating. 'Ananya, be fast. We're kinda in a hurry. Please wrap up whatever you want to say soon.'

She glared at me in dismay. I was a bit rude, but she must have expected that.

'I want to say sorry for my behaviour.'

Not again, I thought to myself. 'It's OK, I told you.'

'No. It's not OK. You have to listen to it all,' she seemed quite determined.

I nodded although I was beginning to tire by then.

'You see, I was just playing around with you all these days.'

As if I didn't know. Anyway, I didn't care anymore. *Las Vegas, casinos and blondes, here I come. Yippee!*

'I was waiting for your call all these days but you didn't call even once.'

'I thought you would be angry with me and it was better that I didn't disturb you and Sachin.'

'Awww!' she frowned. 'It's not like that, maybe I was just pretending to be angry.'

'Everytime?'

'I didn't want you to be around me.'

'Why so?'

'Because I had someone in my life already, Sachin. Why couldn't you just take it casually? Why did you have to fall in love? Why didn't you just fantasize about me like other guys?'

'Well, actually I did but I never showed it,' I grinned sheepishly. She was in splits too.

'I hate this bloody smile of yours,' she pouted and I donned a serious expression. Where was this conversation going, I wondered. I didn't have the least idea but I wasn't enjoying it for sure.

'What now?'

'I don't know,' she shook her head. 'But why can't I stop myself from falling in love with you?'

Did I hear that right? I looked at her in shock.

'I love you,' she said and before I could give her a reaction she fell into my arms.

We hugged.

'Ananya! I'm going to the US tonight,' I said to her.

She stared at me for some time as if doubting it. I nodded to confirm. She smiled.

'That's good! I'm so happy for you,' she pushed me away. Of course, she didn't like the idea of my going away but I had to go, if not for me, then at least for my friends.

'All the best, Gauti,' she gave me a peck on my cheeks.

Damn! How could she do this to me at the last minute! I had waited so long for this moment. I had craved for it and cried for it. I had been ready to die for it. But it came too late. I had changed, I wasn't weak anymore.

⁂

Nineteen hours in a plane is tough, especially when you are sitting in the middle seat. Every time I wanted to go to the loo, the fat aunty sitting next to me made a face. I offered to exchange seats with her but she made a face again, as if I had asked her to strip. I turned to Subho. He seemed excited, sitting in the window seat. Wasn't he tired of seeing the monotonous mighty blue ocean for all those hours? First flight! Or perhaps, that was the first time he might have seen an airport.

I wanted to catch up on sleep but my attempts only made Aunty even more furious. And I just couldn't stop thinking about Ananya, of course. She loved me and I loved her too. So what about our careers? Was it important? I would rather return to handle Dad's business, I thought to myself. I would make more money there than I would anywhere else. But would she be accepted in my family? I could explain to them about her or I could threaten them that I would elope. I could manage it, I was confident about it. And so my thoughts went on and on.

We landed.

They had sent a Hummer to pick us up from the airport. Our jaws dropped to see the gigantic metallic gigantic monster. So we belong to this league now, I thought, beaming with joy. Well, to be frank, that was even my first time in a Hummer. It was like a dream come true. Huge and spacious, the seats were even cozier than those imported couches back home. When we stopped for a drink, I looked inside the bonnet and saw there was an impressive 6.2l V8 diesel engine that powered this monster that measured a full 8 feet in width. It may not be a very practical vehicle, but you can't beat being driven in a Hummer! Moreover, it's a gadget lover's delight—there's even a switch to alter tyre pressure for controlling tyre grip and flotation over soft ground. So if you find yourself driving a Hummer in the desert, you know what to do!

New York had a large Indian population we realized. The top floor of a fifty-storied building had been given to us. I looked around at Subho who had been excited about the swimming pool in our colony back in India, while the apartment we were given had a pool right inside the apartment. There was a small gym too. The Jacuzzi in the bathroom was huge and you could see practically all of New York from the balcony. We had really hit gold.

We were tired and the jet-lag made things a little difficult for us. So for the first day, we stayed indoors instead of exploring the city. After changing, bathing in the pool and calling up family, we got drunk, got stoned and went right off to sleep.

The next day we were informed that the monster would pick us up early the next morning. It was a big day for us, the first day at our new office!

Dreams and Heartbreaks

More than a month passed by and we slowly adapted to our new world. I can confidently say that apart from seeing Moody in mini-skirts and if we ignored the food, life was actually great there. At work, it was even better. Orion Technologies was a small firm of around twenty-four employees, including us. Everyone had their own independent role and was solely responsible for their domain of work. There were no managers and no dim-witted, good-for-nothing, dumb HR staff; we reported directly to our president. Make no mistake, we weren't working for some demanding, disciplined Japanese boss. We worked for Bhupesh Oberoi *(Call me BOB!)*.

To write something about him is the most difficult part of this book. I'm short of words while describing him and missing out on anything about him would be like offending him. Bob. The name suited him just perfectly. Coolness and style reflected in everything he had. He wore almost a kilo of gold, I never saw him in anything but Armani suits, House of Testoni was his chosen brand of shoes and he had made Rolex design an exclusive watch for him. Gosh! And here I thought I was brand-conscious. He was as focused as Narayana Murthy, as sharp as Ratan Tata and as flamboyant as Vijay Mallya. He had come to the US a decade ago and had worked initially as a TV repairman but now owned a Hummer that he used as a cab to pick up his employees whenever they flew in. If not God, he was certainly a demigod to us. Subho even wants to write a biography on him someday.

'Hello, everyone!' He was addressing us after reviewing the first module of our project.

We all greeted him.

'I'll come straight to the point,' he said. We nodded. 'I am very impressed with your work. You guys are just fantastic. The review report is awesome.'

We stole a glance at each other with a little smile; we wanted to scream aloud in joy.

'I'm really impressed. This project will be a revolution. I have decided that you people will be completely responsible for this project, even the client deal part of it,' he continued. We wanted to hug each other right there.

'Moreover, as an appreciation of your dedication and hard work, I make you guys partner for this project. I will handle only the finance and the rest of the credit and rewards will go to your team, even the client part.' He was smiling but it felt as if God was smiling down at us from above. We wanted to drink and get stoned to celebrate our victory.

Bob threw a small party later that night to celebrate the occasion at his place, or should I say, his palace. He had a miniature version of Vegas in his basement, complete with disco lights, a big bar, a dance floor, a terrific music system and a casino where the guests never lost. Bob had made all this with just twenty-two people working with him. Whoa! This man had to be the Alchemist. In reality, we knew of course, that such fortune was only possible in either IT or smuggling.

Though I worshipped him, I have to admit *Bob can't dance saala!* But he wasn't the type to give up easily on anything without even trying, so he hit the floor with the rest of us. I would rate him two on ten for his hilarious dance moves. It was like seeing Donald Duck dance, a fat version, and then joined by his Daisy. Moody. What did you think, she would let the best entrepreneur she had ever met get away? It didn't matter that she was half his age. Our girl was all over him.

But it wasn't just her; everybody seemed to quite like the idea of joining Bob permanently. Everyone except me. I had thought it would be some kind of summer project for a couple of months, we would finish it, earn a lot of money and obtain a certificate of experience that would give us all good jobs back in India. But no, these maniacs wanted to settle there. Subho wanted a green card, Pritam dreamt about joining the US army and flying a Black Hawk, Richa was learning to rap and if rumours are to be believed, Ali actually came to the US to blow away the White House.

'What are you worrying about?' Subho had noticed my restlessness.

'Umm…nothing,' I shrugged.

'Ananya?'

I nodded. Our relationship wasn't going well; a phone call wasn't the same as seeing each other, there was zero momentum, and of course, she was oblivious to Skype.

'You know what, if you get this girl, I will write a book on it,' he said.

I smiled.

'Well bro! I want to share my story with you. The story of the girl whom I always loved. But I couldn't ever explain that to her.'

'Hmm…' I did know a little about her. I had hacked his system, remember?! She was from the US, I recalled. I tuned in to his story with even more interest this time.

'She was with me in high school. I don't know whether it was love at first sight but from whatever I remember of those days, I was in love with her then and I am in love with her now just the same.'

'Does she know?'

He nodded. 'From the beginning itself.'

'Wow! What happened then?'

'Nothing. She had a boyfriend from the A section.'

'And you broke his nose or something,' I laughed but he gave me a cold stare. 'Sorry, jokes apart. So what now?'

'She lives in the US,' he said. I smiled. I knew most of it.

'So, are you going to meet her?'

'Nah!' he shook his head, 'I am not her type.'

'Then what's her type?'

'Well settled, decent family background, big job, lots of money.'

'That's not only her type, it's every girl's type. And anyway why do you worry now? You've got all those qualities. Go and tell her.'

'I don't know. What will I do if she says yes to me?'

I raised one eyebrow. 'What do you mean by that? Marry her.'

'And then…'

'I don't know,' I was confused. 'Take her for a honeymoon. Produce kids.'

'That's it?'

'What else do you want to do?'

'See, when I was in school, I always felt that I wasn't up to the mark for her but I wanted to be. She was popular and I wasn't but I wanted to get there. So I worked hard and topped the class and I became popular but it still wasn't enough. She got into a good college but I couldn't make it because my dad couldn't afford it. I got into engineering as I thought it would make me rich and I tried my hand at everything in college just to be somebody from nobody. She came to the US and now I am following her there too…'

'So, it's all done now. You achieved your goal.'

'That's my point. How do you define a goal? Being human is being greedy for more power, more money and more success. If I get her, I will feel I have achieved everything and relax. Whatever I am today is only because of that craving I had for her and once I have her, all my ambition may just die.'

'But how much more do you want to wait? What about your girl?'

'Maybe until she herself walks up to me,' he said.

I made a face at him, 'Boy, you're so complicated.' He smiled.

And what about me? What was it that I wanted, I wondered.

∞

I took the decision that night itself and didn't tell anybody a thing, knowing I would surely face objection. I wrote a letter about it, placed it on the bed near Subho's pillow and left the room at about three in the morning. The envelope carried my resignation letter too. This time a proper one, not the Muthu kind. And by the time they noticed my absence, I was somewhere near the Middle-East.

When I landed in Mumbai the next day, it was already late evening. The flight was delayed because of heavy rains. I got out of the airport and took a cab to Panvel. But the rains had slowed down the city that always raced ahead of time. It took me nearly four hours in the heavy traffic to reach Ananya's building. I hadn't told her yet about my arrival, I wanted to surprise her. I imagined her reaction when she would open the door and see me standing in front of her. I had left everything behind just to see that reaction.

I rang her doorbell.

'Yes!' her mom opened the door. In my excitement, I had forgotten about this possibility.

I smiled sheepishly. 'Hello, Aunty!'

She looked me up and down. She saw my big bag and probably thought I was a salesman.

'I'm Ananya's colleague,' I clarified.

She looked down at my bag again.

'Well, I was passing by and thought I'd come see her.' I couldn't think of anything else to say. I knew I sounded stupid.

She snapped at me. 'She is out since evening and had called some time ago to inform that she would stay back at Kavita's place.'

'Hmm.'

I walked back down the stairs. I called Ananya many times but her number was switched off. Kavita? She was from Ananya's group at work but I had never talked to her. I called one of the guys I knew in security. I used to give him money to let me smoke in the non-smoking zone.

'Hello Bahadur! This is Gautam.'

'Oh! Hello Sir! How are you?' he greeted me warmly. 'I heard you left the company.'

'Yeah! Dude, I need your help.'

'Tell me Sir.'

'Just get me the number of some Kavita from the accounts department,' I said. 'It will be there in the corporate telebook.'

He searched the telebook and gave me the number.

I called Kavita.

'Hello?'

'Hi! Can I talk to Ananya?'

'What? Who's this?'

'I am...' I paused, wondering what to say. 'I'm her cousin.'

'She is not with me. She went early today; somebody had come to pick her up.'

It didn't take a fraction of a second for me to guess who that somebody would be.

'Was he ugly?'

'What?'

'I mean the guy who picked up Ananya.'

'Yes,' she assumed it was a joke.

Gosh! Sachin? A night out? I felt as if somebody had hit me in the chest, over and over, mercilessly. I walked to the station and sat down on a bench. *She was cheating me? Why?* I felt shattered. There were people moving in all directions around me but I could see nothing. Everything seemed blurred. I just sat there feeling cold. And dead.

That felt like the longest night of my life. The tears just wouldn't stop streaming down my cheeks. My eyes were bloodshot and I had a terrible headache. I was so exhausted that I couldn't even stand up for a minute. I felt as if somebody had broken my limbs and left me there to die.

The station was rather empty for a while during the night break for the locals. The rain stopped around dawn. The station started to fill with people waiting for the first train and then, the first local arrived. The chaos started again.

'Gautam!' Someone put a hand on my shoulder.

I looked up, it was Ananya.

'What you are doing here?' she asked.

I gathered all my energy and stood up. I wanted to face whatever was coming, once and for all.

'Where were you last night?'

'What?'

'Where were you, Ananya?'

'What's wrong with you?'

'Sachin?'

She was astonished. 'What do you mean?'

'A night out with him, you finally did it, right?'

'Shut up, Gautam! Are you mad?'

'Why did you spend a night with him then?'

'Listen Gautam...you know nothing about it.'

'Then tell me Ananya. I've been waiting here all night just to know the reason. Why Ananya? Wasn't my love enough for you?'

Silence.

I could see tears welling up in her eyes but that weapon was now futile. I was not to be carried away this time. I wanted my answers.

'Tell me Ananya. Tell me,' I demanded.

'I don't think I need to justify myself. Moreover, you're not in a condition to understand. We will talk later,' and she started to walk.

'No Ananya. We are not going to talk again. It's over. I don't want to see you again in my life.'

She didn't stop and walked slowly to the overbridge. That baffled me even further and I shouted after her.

'You're a bitch.'

That Thing Called Love

Two years had gone by since that day and here I was, waiting for her at the airport. All my efforts to move on had been in vain. I had returned to the US and joined Bob. I never visited India in that period; my parents visited me thrice but were unable to convince me to return to India. I had worked really hard to earn the nicknames 'Dumb Developer' and 'Mad Boxer'. Now I had a flight to catch in an hour and I prayed that she was delayed. I regretted calling her; I didn't really want to see her again. I mean what would I say to her. She was probably someone's wife by now, she must have married that snob Sachin. I imagined her, wearing geeky old-fashioned glasses, with a few wrinkles on her face, extra pounds on her waistline, in a sari, with a typical hairstyle and maybe a child clinging to her. It was scary.

There was the first announcement for the passengers of my flight to proceed to boarding. She wouldn't make it; I felt relief and walked towards the terminal.

'Gautam!' That was Ananya, for sure.

I turned around. No sari but a salwar kameez, the same hairstyle and a leaner figure, but there was a little girl with her. Heartbreak.

'Ananya!' I waved at her. I feared Sachin might be around too somewhere.

'You seem to be in a hurry,' she said as she reached me. There was a pleasant smile on her face. Did she forget that the last time we met, I had called her a bitch?

'Not really.'

'How are you?'

'I'm fine.' I looked at her closely. No *mangalsutra*. No *sindoor*.

But that child, she was cute. *Sachin's? I had my doubts.*

'So, how is everything? I mean your life, husband and all…' I asked her straight off. I had had enough of the suspense.

'Let me guess, you think this child is mine?'

Wasn't it? I made a face.

'Gauti! She is five years old. Can't you see? She is my neighbour's child; her mom left her with me because she had to go out.' She slapped her forehead in an overdramatic manner.

I was stumped. I didn't want to prod further. It didn't really matter to me anymore. I just wanted to run away.

'What about you?' she asked.

'Umm…nothing. I an getting late. I have to go now. Nice to see you, Ananya.' I pulled my bag closer. Subho was waiting for me inside.

'Wait,' she held my hand. 'You can't go this time.'

'Why shouldn't I?'

'Because you need to know something about that night.'

I looked at her stunned.

'Gauti, I did go to meet Sachin that night.'

'I guess I know that.' This was getting worse. I desperately wanted Subho to come out and take me away.

'Gautam! I didn't sleep with him that night.'

I was aghast. 'Whatever. I don't care. Why are you telling me this now?'

'Because I love you damn it! That's what I went to tell him that evening.'

'What?' I stared at her. She sat on a nearby chair, covering her face with her palms, she was about to sob. The little child gave me a stern look.

'Anu! I'm sorry,' I sat down beside her. 'Tell me everything.'

She looked at me, the tears had already started flowing. I wiped them with my hand. She smiled a little.

'After you went to the US, Sachin started pushing me for marriage and I wanted to tell him about you. That night he had asked me out on a date and I thought I'd tell him everything. So I did. And he was angry and left me as I had expected. I never saw him again. While returning home I got stuck in the rain so I called my mom and lied to her about Kavita. I returned by the first train next morning and met you at the station.'

'What? Why didn't you tell me all this that day?'

'Did you let me say anything?'

'But…'

'I thought you wouldn't have believed me anyway. I thought it was a test of my love. I always knew if my love for you was true, you would definitely return to me.'

'Two years, Ananya?' I couldn't believe she could be that stupid or was it actually I who was the stupid one?

'Was it my fault? You disappeared. I didn't have your number. You blocked me on Facebook, email, wherever possible. I had no other option but to just wait for you.'

I wondered how to react? I had spent two years hating the girl I loved and punishing myself for no reason. I looked down, I couldn't face her.

'Gautam! I am thirty-one. Will you please marry me?' she said with a little smile.

So what was I supposed to do? Apologize? Ask Subho? Run away? My brain went into airplane mode. No more thinking. It was now up to my heart. I smiled back at her and took her into my arms. We kissed. And that was only our second kiss.

∽

Yeah I missed the flight. We got married. How? That's another big story. Anyway, we went to the US and settled down there. Dad now has a branch of his finance company in New York, headed by Ananya. I am doing well, I am now among the directors at Orion Technologies and why not, since Moody is the CEO. She married Bob. She also hunted down Samir and broke his leg. Subho, they say, is dating Lacie Heart. Pritam finally gave up hopes on Moody and joined ISKCON. Richa hooked up with a German guy from the rap band; she now has the fairest husband in her whole village history and is quite happy flaunting it. Ali too was in love, yeah! With the same guy of Richa's but he has now moved on. Together, we work for Orion Technologies which now has over five thousand employees worldwide and was also listed in the New York stock exchange a few months ago.

So there…that is the story of a few IT nerds who finally made their dreams come true and lived happily ever after.

And oh yeah…Coming soon…Three months from now, Armaan will be here!

Acknowledgements

I grew in a society where most parents want their children to grow up to be engineers. On my graduation day, I still remember, when my principal asked me what does this engineering degree means to me, I had a fair idea of the reply he expected from me—bright future, successful career, respectable job, high status and stable life. But I smiled at him and said, 'It means freedom to me.' But then, how long could this priced freedom last? I had only twenty days in hand before I joined my first job. Just twenty days of my own in return of the twenty years I spent in school and college. But, at least now I won't have to study anymore, I consoled myself. But hang on! Wasn't I in IT where you need to study until you retire or die? And, the big challenges were yet to come—office politics, ratings, IT returns, clients, night shifts and bugs. 'Give me some sunshine, give me some rain…' This is how I felt after spending two years in the corporate.

An engineer on the weekdays and an author on weekends—it's really tough to handle. No holidays, no pubs, no parties and no girlfriend, I actually had no life. But then, my friends and my fans were always with me and here's the result of their support—*IT Hurts*. I thank all of them for motivating me and keeping me going in testing times. Anubhav, Chhanda, Mayuri, Parul, Prity, Priyanka, Pushpendra, Shrestha, Sovik, Swagata, Soumyorup, Tara and Udita, you all did more than just following me on Social Networking sites. Abhishek, Ajay, Misbah, Rohan, Sandeep, Shravan, Sudeep and Ujjwal; I know you jerks don't care about this and I love you all for that. A special thanks to Ankur, Bhupesh and Ravi, my office colleagues, for helping me with codes to IT returns forms. Rajashree, Rashmi Kumar, Shikha

Sharma and Tuhin Sinha, my fellow writers who were always there to help whenever I needed, thank you very much.

And finally a very big thanks to Mahi Singla, my pretty co-author. On our first meeting I told her I couldn't complete *IT Hurts* because I was busy preparing for CAT. She was disappointed to know that like others I too chose to be a corporate slave instead of chasing my dreams. I laughed and asked her to complete the rest of the story. And six months later we signed up the contract for *IT Hurts*. She owns this book more than me.

My heartfelt thank you to my publishers Rupa Publications for giving me another opportunity to be a part of their list which also includes my hero Chetan Bhagat.

Last but not the least, a big applause for my readers for their love and appreciation. Those fan mails make my day guys, so please keep them coming in. Cheers!

www.ingramcontent.com/pod-product-compliance
Lightning Source LLC
Chambersburg PA
CBHW020610270326
41927CB00005B/258